Practicing Medicine and Ethics

To practice medicine and ethics, physicians need wisdom and integrity to integrate scientific knowledge, patient preferences, their own moral commitments, and society's expectations. This work of integration requires that a physician pursue certain goals of care, determine moral priorities, and understand that conscience or integrity requires harmony among a person's beliefs, values, reasoning, actions, and identity. But the moral and religious pluralism of contemporary society makes this integration challenging and uncertain. How physicians treat patients will depend on the particular beliefs and values they and other health professionals bring to each instance of shared decision making. This book offers a framework for practical wisdom in medicine that addresses the need for integrity in the life of each health professional. In doing so, it acknowledges the challenge of moral pluralism and the need for moral dialogue and humility as professionals fulfill their obligations to patients, themselves, and society.

Lauris Christopher Kaldjian is Director of the Program in Bioethics and Humanities at the University of Iowa Carver College of Medicine, where he holds the Richard M. Caplan Chair in Biomedical Ethics and Medical Humanities and is also a professor in the Department of Internal Medicine. His research interests have been directed toward end-of-life concerns, goals of care, disclosure of medical errors, ethics education, and the role of philosophical and religious beliefs in clinical decision making. He has received research grants from the Robert Wood Johnson Foundation and the John Templeton Foundation, and his publications can be found in a variety of medical and bioethics journals. At the University of Iowa Hospitals and Clinics, he practices outpatient general internal medicine, chairs the Ethics Committee, and serves as Medical Director for Clinical Ethics. In the College of Medicine, he teaches ethics to medical students and co-directs the Humanities Distinction Track. He has served on the Ethics Committee of the United Network for Organ Sharing, chaired the Ethics Committee of the Society of General Internal Medicine, and served as a deputy editor of the *Journal of General Internal Medicine.* He currently chairs the Committee on Law and Ethics of the Iowa Medical Society. He is a member of the American Society of Bioethics and Humanities and a Fellow of the American College of Physicians.

Practicing Medicine and Ethics

Integrating Wisdom, Conscience, and Goals of Care

LAURIS CHRISTOPHER KALDJIAN
University of Iowa

CAMBRIDGE
UNIVERSITY PRESS

CAMBRIDGE
UNIVERSITY PRESS

32 Avenue of the Americas, New York, NY 10013-2473, USA

Cambridge University Press is part of the University of Cambridge.

It furthers the University's mission by disseminating knowledge in the pursuit of education, learning, and research at the highest international levels of excellence.

www.cambridge.org
Information on this title: www.cambridge.org/9781107012165

First published 2014

Printed in the United States of America

A catalog record for this publication is available from the British Library.

Library of Congress Cataloging in Publication Data
Kaldjian, Lauris Christopher, 1963–
Practicing medicine and ethics : integrating wisdom, conscience, and goals of care / Lauris Christopher Kaldjian.
pages cm
Includes bibliographical references and index.
ISBN 978-1-107-01216-5 (hardback)
1. Medical ethics. 2. Integrity. 3. Humility. I. Title.
R724.K295 2014
174.2–dc23 2013049178

ISBN 978-1-107-01216-5 Hardback

For Heather and Anna

Contents

Acknowledgments

In the course of writing this book, I have incurred many debts of gratitude. The idea of crafting my interests in medicine and ethics within a framework of wisdom was sparked by the Defining Wisdom Project, an endeavor sponsored by the University of Chicago and funded by the John Templeton Foundation. A grant from this project provided financial support from 2008 to 2010, as well as a warm, engaging, and interdisciplinary community of scholars. My efforts were also assisted by a Career Development Award from the University of Iowa that provided time for writing during the summers of 2009 and 2010. Beatrice Rehl at Cambridge University Press graciously received me unannounced at her office in New York in 2010, and her immediate interest in the topic of this book came as a great encouragement at a key juncture. As each chapter makes clear, I have borrowed many insights from many authors. The extent of my appreciation for their contributions to my understanding is reflected in the frequency of citations throughout the text. Though all weaknesses and missteps in this book are my own, their number and severity have been diminished by the generous efforts of three colleagues who reviewed an earlier version of the entire manuscript. Gene Outka – one of my mentors in ethics when I was at Yale and renowned for his work in philosophical and theological ethics – graciously accepted this task of review when his own writing projects should have kept him from doing so. Thomas Duffy – my mentor in medicine at Yale and the personification of integrity in the life of a physician – applied his diagnostic skills to strengthen areas of need. Donald Dacey – a devoted friend and man of keen insights – lavished far too many hours engaging in dialogue over each chapter, providing critical feedback that winnowed, clarified, and sharpened the text and content. The process of refining continued through Mary Becker's excellent attention to detail as a copy editor. My parents, Movses and Maija Kaldjian, faithfully encouraged my efforts and continued to teach me what it means to love in sickness and in health. My debt is greatest to those who are nearest. Anna, my daughter, lovingly accepted the burdens of having a father who had to tend to "the book" during hours that we could have spent playing more violin duets. Heather, my wife and fellow traveler on this and all journeys, could not have been more selfless in her commitment, assistance, encouragement, and love. My debt here is truly immeasurable. *Sola Dei gratia.*

Preface

To practice medicine and ethics, physicians need wisdom and integrity. These characteristics allow physicians to integrate the wide range of information and values that arise from scientific knowledge, patient preferences, their own moral commitments, and society's expectations. Learning to bring these domains together is an essential part of becoming a physician, and it determines the ethics that guides the care of patients.

The integration of these domains may seem obvious and effortless when medical practice proceeds smoothly on widely shared notions of health, health care, and professional standards. But the practice of medicine includes ethical challenges that arise from serious moral uncertainties and disagreements that disturb what might otherwise look like a calm sea of consensus. These challenges are exacerbated by the diversity of moral beliefs, values, and frameworks that pervade society and the medical profession. The moral pluralism created by these differences means that decision making shared by patients and physicians is influenced by an interplay of moral values that may include significant contrasts that create tensions and conflicts. Physicians need practical wisdom and integrity to navigate this morally diverse landscape and make ethics a meaningful part of shared decision making. Without wisdom and integrity, physicians will be at a loss to perceive, adjudicate between, and reconcile the competing moral claims that can arise during the process of clinical decision making – a process that fundamentally depends on the beliefs and values of the persons participating in it.

Some may assume that the medical profession cultivates wisdom and integrity among its members by promoting medical ethics. This assumption should be questioned in light of the variable ways medical ethics may be taught and discussed. Common approaches readily refer to technologies to be assessed, values to be considered, and persons to be respected – but they may miss what practical wisdom requires: that we must identify the *ends* worth pursuing through medicine before we can appropriately decide which medical *means* should be employed. Instead of identifying such ends, medical ethics typically moves quickly to discussions about guiding principles, likely consequences, and procedures to be followed in the absence of consensus about which principles and consequences should be given highest priority.

The ethics that tends to dominate the medical profession may also struggle with or neglect to reconcile different *approaches* to ethical reasoning, leaving some persons – especially reflective medical trainees – to wonder how they are supposed to find a way to weave together different sources of ethical value into a meaningful whole. Current renditions of medical ethics may also give insufficient attention to the contrasting *responsibilities* a physician experiences – to patients, to herself, and to society. In situations where these responsibilities are in tension or conflict, how is a physician supposed to proceed? How, for instance, is she supposed to reconcile respect for patient autonomy with concern for her own integrity or her obligations to society?

The need to reconcile different approaches and responsibilities points to the importance of the integration that practical wisdom entails. This kind of integration lies at the center of the framework for practical wisdom offered in this book, a framework that reaches back to the tradition of virtue ethics so that we can understand what ethics in medicine should encompass and what practical wisdom should mean. Virtue ethics focuses attention on moral ends; as a result, its relevance may be questionable in settings where consensus about moral ends is lacking. In medicine, however, virtue ethics carries considerable potential, since health-related goals – such as curing disease and providing comfort – enjoy broad consensus. The virtue of practical wisdom is of special relevance to medicine because it promotes practical responses that combine objective assessment and moral evaluation through deliberation focused on ends.

The essential role that ends play in virtue ethics reminds us that good decision making always has a goal in view, a goal that is presumed to be good and worthy of pursuit. Virtue ethics also points to character and motivation as essential complements to moral reasoning, and the relationship between moral character and moral reasoning invites careful consideration of integrity in the moral life. To gain a better understanding of integrity, this book explores the meaning of conscience and finds enough overlap between the two concepts to recommend that conscience and integrity be treated as interchangeable labels for a single moral domain.

One of the dimensions of this domain is moral reasoning. This rational dimension has great implications for medicine and ethics, since it allows conscience or integrity to span the moral space between persons through moral dialogue. Another aspect of this domain is integration, an idea nicely embedded in the word *integrity*, indicating the need for a wholeness in the moral life that unifies beliefs, values, and actions. This need pushes against any suggestions that a physician's life can be split or compartmentalized into personal and professional domains.

The framework for practical wisdom offered in these pages centers on integrity as it reflects a person's need to harmonize the moral beliefs and values he holds to be important for making a decision. The framework also centers on integrity by reflecting a person's need to take responsibility for his own actions related to a decision. All persons are responsible for the ethics by which they act, and to take responsibility for an action is, in a sense, to authorize it on the basis of beliefs and values that reside at the center of integrity. Because it focuses on the moral lives of individuals in these ways, the framework proposed here is appropriately described as *integrity-centered.*

The problem of moral pluralism and its implications for medicine and ethics are pervasive themes in this book. Practical wisdom in medicine depends on the moral beliefs and values that clinicians bring to their professional work, and these beliefs and values will inevitably encounter what is, more or less, a pluralistic moral environment. How should physicians address moral differences among persons participating in shared decision making? What kinds of personal resources, interpersonal processes, and social arrangements may help facilitate shared decision making, professional cooperation, and conflict resolution in the midst of moral diversity? Can there be a morally neutral vantage point by which all parties in a decision can assume an objective perspective? The challenges of practicing medicine in a morally pluralistic setting invite us to wrestle with these questions.

Communication is another important theme, because it is essential to shared decision making and one of the most basic ways in which clinicians show respect for their patients. To communicate routine medical information accurately and understandably is challenging enough, but how and when should physicians communicate about the moral beliefs and values they rely on to guide decision making? Does communication about such beliefs and values benefit patients or physicians, or both? Should we expect someone who makes a conscience-based moral claim to communicate the moral reasons behind that claim? Can moral dialogue within a professional community help physicians calibrate their moral assessments in light of each other's moral assumptions, priorities, and practices? These types of questions arise as we consider the ethical importance of communication as a means of respecting others by explaining the reasons that motivate and justify our actions.

As a physician-ethicist at an academic medical center, I am involved in teaching, research, and patient care. In my clinical work I practice general internal medicine, which is sometimes referred to as primary care for adults. Because of my background in medicine, I take special interest in the needs and responsibilities of physicians. That said, the issues addressed in this book are relevant to all health professionals. Nurses, physician assistants, pharmacists, and others have the same needs as physicians for an integrated approach to clinical care and ethics, even if their role-specific responsibilities differ. To acknowledge this broad relevance, I sometimes use inclusive categories, such as *clinician* and *health professional*, as the occupational frame of reference.

I hope the concerns addressed in this book will be of interest to health professionals, ethicists, educators, administrators, and persons involved in health policy. I also hope these issues will be meaningful to people without a formal background in health care but who are nevertheless interested in how health care decisions are made and how moral beliefs and values influence those decisions. All of us are or will be patients, and we should consider how the beliefs and values of our health care providers affect the care we and our loved ones receive.

It may help the reader if I explain briefly how this book is organized. Its ten chapters can be divided into four parts. The first part comprises Chapters 1–3. Together they provide a backdrop describing medicine as a goal-directed moral practice, virtue ethics as a vitally important way of understanding what moral resources health professionals need for participating in that practice, and practical wisdom as an ancient virtue with direct contemporary relevance to clinical decision making. The second part comprises Chapters 4–6. Drawing from ancient and modern sources, they present conscience as a multidimensional way of understanding what matters most in the moral life; moral integrity as a matter of integrating beliefs, values, reasoning, actions, and identity; and grounds for viewing conscience and integrity as largely interchangeable. Chapters 7–9 make up the third part and address the significance of moral integrity for health professionals in light of the moral and religious pluralism that marks Western society and medical practice. The last part is Chapter 10. It draws from the preceding nine chapters to offer an integrity-centered framework for practical wisdom in medicine, suggest ways of fostering practical wisdom amid moral pluralism, and illustrate some of the implications of practical wisdom for clinical practice. To assist the reader, I provide summaries at the end of each of the first nine chapters. Those who prefer to proceed quickly to the framework for practical wisdom can use these nine summaries as abbreviated stepping stones to Chapter 10.

To aspire to practical wisdom in medicine is a great goal. It is also a great challenge, due to the personal demands of acquiring a valuable skill and the moral cross-currents of a pluralistic society. Meeting this challenge requires a constellation of attitudes and habits that promote careful observation, clear reasoning, respectful communication, goals of care, and abiding moral commitments. It requires us to acknowledge the foundational beliefs and values that drive our thinking, speaking, and acting. And it invites us to consider the interdependence between wisdom, integrity, and identity. If we neglect these concerns, ethics will be uprooted from the moral foundations that reflect what each of us holds, at the end of the day, to be real and good. Such neglect does no one a service. But if we engage these concerns, we will be in a better position to understand what wisdom and integrity mean for shared decision making in medicine and how vital they are for health professionals and the patients they serve.

1

Medicine as a Goal-Directed, Moral Practice

Physicians and other health care professionals face many challenging decisions, and for this reason they need practical wisdom. Practical wisdom is a virtue, or character trait, that allows those who have it to respond well to a challenge of decision making – that is, to respond with realistic appreciation for the objective features of a situation and with sensitivity to the moral values it involves. Practical wisdom is ends-oriented, which is to say that knowledge of what *ends* are worth pursuing ought to precede consideration of what *means* are most likely to achieve those ends. Because practical wisdom is directed toward an end, it is a purpose-driven pursuit, one that seeks the best means to fulfill an end or achieve a goal. In the absence of ends or goals, practical wisdom ceases to carry the meaning it otherwise implies. As an ends-oriented virtue, practical wisdom is therefore *teleological* because it is directed toward, and guided by, an end (in Greek, *telos*). The relationship between wisdom and ends is of central importance in this book, and to understand what practical wisdom means in medicine, we must first understand what the practice of medicine accepts as its ends or goals. In Chapter 3, practical wisdom will be discussed in much more detail.

I. INTERNAL AND EXTERNAL GOODS RELATED TO MEDICAL PRACTICE

Any discussion of medicine's ends will reveal that there is wide agreement about what kinds of goals the practice of medicine should pursue. But if discussions probe deeply and broadly enough, it will also become apparent that people disagree about some of the goals that may be associated with the practice of medicine. One source of disagreement stems from divergent beliefs about whether the goals of medicine are properly viewed as intrinsic or extrinsic to the practice of medicine itself. *Intrinsic ends* concern those aspects of medical practice that relate most closely, and respond most directly, to the human experience of illness and the bodily and mental effects of disease. Medicine's intrinsic ends would include the well-known goals of healing, comforting, and preventing disease – ends that are so easily taken for granted that it may seem strange to suggest they could be otherwise. These intrinsic ends may be said to represent the *internal goods* of medical practice, on the grounds that these goods are inseparable from the practice of medicine as we currently understand it. The claim that such goods are internal implies that their validity is independent of, and prior to, other considerations such as professional standards, patient preferences, public policies, social conventions, and historical circumstances.

By contrast, *extrinsic ends* concern those uses to which medicine may be put in the service of goals that do not relate directly to purposes such as healing, comfort, and disease prevention. Extrinsic ends correspond to other goals that justify and guide medical activity. Examples of extrinsic ends in medical practice are not hard to find. A team physician can use his skills to stabilize an athlete's injury and minimize her pain in order to enhance her team's prospects for victory. A general internist can perform a physical examination and laboratory testing to determine a prospective employee's health insurance risks. A psychiatrist can determine an accused person's competence to stand trial. A military physician can use vaccinations to enhance national security by lessening soldiers' vulnerability to biological agents of warfare. A pediatrician can prescribe growth hormone to treat a young boy's short stature and thus improve – according to parental estimations – his prospects in life. Such examples illustrate how extrinsic ends arise from circumstances, preferences, or priorities that motivate people and organizations to employ medicine as a means to ends other than, or beyond, direct healing, comfort, or disease prevention for individual patients.

The distinction between intrinsic and extrinsic ends, or internal and external goods, has both advocates and critics. One advocate, Edmund Pellegrino, argues that the basis for the distinction is real and vital, maintaining that the ends of medicine can and should be derived from values internal to medicine (what he calls the *essentialist* position) rather than from values externally imposed on medicine by society (what he calls the *socially constructed* position). The essentialist position derives its ends from the nature of medicine itself, whereas the socially constructed position derives its ends from an external social source "arrived at by social dialogue, consensus formation, political process, or negotiation."[1] With colleague David Thomasma, Pellegrino offers a phenomenological justification for an essentialist position within a philosophy of medicine that provides a teleological account of medical practice based on its internal goods.[2] Within this account, the ends of curing, caring, helping, and healing form a valid *telos* of medicine because these ends are derived from the internal goods of medicine. But conceptions of medical practice based on traditional notions of internal goods have their critics. Those who view the practice of medicine as a socially constructed enterprise offer a competing perspective, claiming that medicine's social organization is more determinative than its proposed philosophical foundations or perceived ethical norms, at least as far as predicting the behavior of medical professionals is concerned.[3]

In contrast to the essentialist and socially constructed views, a third alternative can be called the *professionally constructed* perspective, according to which professionals impose their own values on the practice of medicine. This view suggests that medical professionals are the authors of their own practice, that they develop and maintain their own concepts of health and disease, which are value-loaded rather than scientifically objective, and that they use these concepts to justify and achieve professionally determined goals. Critics of a professionally constructed perspective of medicine may offer contrasting views in which patients and physicians are supposed to negotiate the terms of the medical encounter. One such approach recommends that patients bring to medical professionals any problem that concerns them and then negotiate the terms of interpreting the problem in a way that allows both the patient and the professional to participate in the process of interpretation. One advocate of this approach claims that, after such dialogue, "a patient is usually quite ready to change his view of what his problem is from purely a symptomatic one to one that ties the symptoms, present and possible, to a disease, and the physician, for his part, is often quite ready to adapt his notion of a problem, diagnosed in terms of a particular disease, to what it will mean to

[1] Edmund D. Pellegrino, "The goals and ends of medicine: how are they to be defined?" in *Physician & philosopher: the philosophical foundation of medicine – essays by Dr. Edmund Pellegrino*, ed. Roger J. Bulger and John P. McGovern (Charlottesville, VA: Carden Jennings, 2001), 59.

[2] Edmund D. Pellegrino and David C. Thomasma, *A philosophical basis of medical practice: toward a philosophy and ethic of the healing professions* (New York: Oxford University Press, 1981).

[3] Eliot Freidson, *Profession of medicine: a study of the sociology of applied knowledge* (Chicago: University of Chicago Press, 1970), 5.

the patient in the short run and in the long run."[4] On such an account, the practice of medicine is a process of consensus about what is allowed to count as a medical problem, and the patient–clinician relationship is an interpretive partnership that is entitled to make this determination.

Given the predictive powers and interventional techniques that have been achieved through biomedical science and clinical investigation, some may find it strange that anyone would suggest that patients ought to be empowered to influence the definition of what constitutes a medical problem. They might suggest that a more objective status should be granted to the patient–physician encounter, one that is less dependent on the subjective perspectives of patients and professionals. But critics of professionally constructed views of medicine are right to draw our attention to the ways in which subjective values can affect how our concepts of health and disease are defined and how goals of medicine are derived from these concepts. Such critics also remind us of the importance of patient–physician dialogues that acknowledge and engage the particular beliefs and needs of patients, without denying the validity of the knowledge and skill that professionals gain from training in biomedical science and through clinical experience.

II. DIVERGENT CONCEPTS OF HEALTH AND DISEASE

Unsettling as they may be, questions about the degree to which medicine is an objective endeavor encourage us to examine assumptions that may be embedded in our basic concepts. Common meanings of *health* and *disease* are largely taken for granted in the practice of medicine, by physicians and patients alike, and we do not usually pause to discuss their meanings when we hear phrases such as "Smoking is bad for your *health*," "Cardiovascular *diseases* kill many Americans," "the National Institutes of *Health*," "the Department of Public *Health*," or "the Centers for *Disease* Control and Prevention." Indeed, it would be a rare event to hear a patient and physician discuss the meanings of health or disease during a clinical encounter. But these observations about common practice should not cause us to conclude that consideration of the meanings of our basic concepts is unimportant.

4 John Ladd, "The internal morality of medicine: an essential dimension of the patient–physician relationship," in *The clinical encounter*, ed. Earl E. Shelp (Dordrecht: Reidel, 1983), 228.

Questions prompted by philosophical, historical, and sociological observations readily reveal the extent to which the meanings of health and disease can be debated and how their various interpretations carry implications for the way medicine is conceptualized and practiced. Consider, for example, how concepts of disease have evolved over thousands of years, with competition between perspectives that view disease as a reality existing separately from the persons it affects and perspectives that view disease as a deviation from whatever society considers normal.[5] In addition to the fascinating variability in the way diseases have been classified (nosology) from one historical period to another, observers also point out how values are active in identifying undesirable conditions (that are judged bad and are therefore considered diseases) and desirable conditions (that are judged good and are therefore considered manifestations of health). Such observations support the conclusion that concepts of health and disease are determined by a mixture of scientific, statistical, and cultural norms, resulting in a definition of disease as "the aggregate of those conditions which, judged by the prevailing culture, are deemed painful, or disabling, and which, at the same time, deviate from either the statistical norm or from some idealized status."[6] By correlation, health is the absence of disease.

But not everyone agrees that concepts of health and disease are derived only from some mixture of scientific, statistical, and cultural norms. Leon Kass, for example, observes that the English and Greek origins of terms pertaining to health signify "wholeness" (English, *health*) and "living well" (Greek, *hygeia*) and that these terms have a standing that exists independent of their linguistic associations with disease.[7] His Aristotelian conclusion is that health is "the well working of the organism as a whole" and this "well working" is a natural norm characterized by specific excellences of the human body,[8] not a value judgment imposed by a society or culture onto a "value-neutral condition of the body."[9] H. Tristram Engelhardt offers an assessment that resonates with Kass's view by suggesting that health serves as a unifying regulative ideal that represents the common

5 Henry Cohen, "The evolution of the concept of disease," in *Concepts of health and disease: interdisciplinary perspectives*, ed. Arthur L. Caplan, H. Tristram Engelhardt, and James J. McCartney (London: Addison-Wesley, 1981), 209–19.

6 Lester S. King, "What is disease?" in *Concepts of health and disease*, ed. Caplan et al., 112.

7 Leon R. Kass, "Regarding the end of medicine and the pursuit of health," in *Concepts of health and disease*, ed. Caplan et al., 15.

8 Ibid., 18.

9 Ibid., 13.

direction away from all the various diseases. However, he differs from Kass in holding that both disease and health are simultaneously descriptive *and* normative concepts, as both involve explanation and evaluation.[10] In contrast to the approaches of Kass and Engelhardt, a sociological perspective of health may focus on the individual's ability to participate in society, as evidenced by Talcott Parsons's description of health as "the state of optimum *capacity* of an individual for the effective performance of the roles and tasks for which he has been socialized."[11]

For the purposes of this book, I acknowledge the shifting currents of nosology in the history of medicine and the normative implications for medical practice of the malleability of the concept of disease. But with Kass, I also assume that health has an objective aspect that need not be in conflict with its subjective interpretation and experience for individual patients.[12] I further assume with Parsons that there are features of health and illness that are common to all human beings on the basis of their shared constitutions, features that would also be expected to vary as a function of social and cultural circumstances.[13] Finally, I acknowledge the implications of George Engel's warnings against reducing health and illness to a set of narrow biomedical parameters, as well as his call for a biopsychosocial model of illness that takes account of the multidimensional ways in which the biological substratum of disease affects and is affected by an individual's psychological, behavioral, and social contexts.[14] Together, these assumptions constitute a perspective that recognizes objective features of human biology, subjective features of human valuing, and contextual features of human society.

Our diverse concepts of health and disease, and the extent to which their meanings are believed to be either objectively verifiable or socially constructed, indicate why the goals of medicine can be viewed as having an intrinsic or extrinsic justification. Significant implications flow from these divergent sources of justification and their potentially contrasting values. The importance of this intrinsic–extrinsic dichotomy was

[10] H. Tristram Engelhardt, "The concepts of health and disease," in *Concepts of health and disease*, ed. Caplan et al., 31–43.

[11] Talcott Parsons, "Definitions of health and illness in the light of American values and social structure," in *Concepts of health and disease*, ed. Caplan et al., 69.

[12] Kass, "Regarding the end of medicine and the pursuit of health," 12.

[13] Parsons, "Definitions of health and illness in the light of American values and social structure," 57, 61, 62.

[14] George L. Engel, "The need for a new medical model: a challenge for biomedicine," in *Concepts of health and disease*, ed. Caplan et al., 589–607.

addressed by a group of international scholars convened by the Hastings Center to identify goals that should guide the practice of medicine.[15] They labeled the two sides of this dichotomy the *inherentist* and *social construction* views. The inherentist position holds that "medicine's proper ends are constituted as a response intrinsic in medicine's practice to the universal human experience of illness."[16] By contrast, the social construction position holds that the great variability of medicine's goals over time and across cultures – due to variable interpretations of disease, illness, and health – makes it difficult to identify a single set of inherent values that would determine a common and enduring set of goals. Medicine on this view is seen as "an evolving fund of knowledge and a changing range of clinical practices that have no fixed essence" and are characterized by "scientific and social malleability."[17] Notably, these scholars were unable to achieve full consensus on whether the goals of medicine should be derived from inherent features of medical practice or from socially constructed features. Instead, they affirmed both perspectives, concluding that "medicine has essential ends, shaped by more or less universal ideals and kinds of historical practices, but its knowledge and skills also lend themselves to a significant degree of social construction."[18] They also believed, however, that the medical profession should rely on its historical traditions and its "inner direction and core values" in order to avoid being misused by society.[19]

Acknowledging the need to come to terms with questions about our concepts of health and disease is an important first step in appreciating how our understanding of medicine as a moral practice depends on beliefs about what medicine's purposes should be. Practical wisdom in medicine depends fundamentally on goals derived from these purposes. An understanding of practical wisdom in medicine will be shared only to the extent that there is consensus about medicine's goals. Before discussing specific goals considered appropriate for medicine, it will be helpful to pursue a bit further the question of medicine's internal features by appropriating insights from Alasdair MacIntyre's analysis of the relationship between virtues and the notion of a *practice*. In the process, the

[15] Mark J. Hanson and Daniel Callahan, eds., *The goals of medicine: the forgotten issues in health care reform* (Washington, DC: Georgetown University Press, 1999).

[16] Ibid., 15.

[17] Ibid., 16.

[18] Ibid.

[19] Ibid.

difference between medicine's internally and externally derived goods, or ends, will become clearer.

III. MEDICINE AS A PRACTICE AND THE POTENTIAL FOR TENSION BETWEEN INTERNAL AND EXTERNAL GOODS

In *After Virtue*, MacIntyre describes moral virtue as it relates to the concept of a *practice* and the way in which different goods, or ends, may be internal or external to a practice. His definition of a practice is, admittedly, not simple: "any coherent and complex form of socially established cooperative human activity through which goods internal to that form of activity are realized in the course of trying to achieve those standards of excellence which are appropriate to, and partially definitive of, that form of activity, with the result that human powers to achieve excellence, and human conceptions of the ends and goods involved, are systematically extended."[20] The length and substance of this definition indicate how significant a human endeavor a practice is, on this view. And if one reads this definition with health care in mind, it is not hard to see how directly it applies to the practice of medicine.

For MacIntyre, internal goods are a necessary feature of a practice and a prerequisite for understanding how virtue functions in the context of a practice. The ability to recognize the internal goods of a practice is gained by participating in that practice, such that those who lack the relevant experience are incompetent to judge a practice's internal goods.[21] Moreover, because a practice involves standards of excellence and obedience to rules, those who enter a practice necessarily submit their professional performance and attitudes to the authority of those standards.[22] Finally, the achievement of the internal goods of a practice is not the individual accomplishment of an independent practitioner, but rather represents a success for all who participate in that practice.[23] On MacIntyre's account, medical practice entails an intimate relationship between the internal goods pursued by individual professionals to the benefit of patients – such as healing, comfort, and disease prevention – and the overall good that sustains the community of medical professionals.

[20] Alasdair MacIntyre, *After virtue* (Notre Dame, IN: University of Notre Dame Press, 1984), 187.
[21] Ibid., 189–90.
[22] Ibid., 190.
[23] Ibid., 190–91.

There is therefore an interdependence between the internal goods, the individuals who make up the community of practice, and the community of practice itself. Such an account places the question of medicine's internal goods at the center of any discussion of how virtue ethics and practical wisdom should be understood in medicine.

To view the medical profession as a community of practice – in which internal goods are definitive and standards of excellence authoritative – is to view medical professionals as members of a moral community who are defined not only by a technical practice, but also by ethical standards that are constitutive of their professional identity. MacIntyre's account relates *practice* to *ethics* by defining virtues as those qualities of professionals that are essential to achieve the internal goods of a practice.[24] Virtues – such as compassion, benevolence, justice, courage, and honesty – not only shape the character of interactions between medical professionals and patients, but also are the means by which professionals define their relationships to each other.

MacIntyre distinguishes between internal and external goods to draw a contrast between *practices* and the *institutions* that sustain them. As an illustration of this internal–external distinction, consider in medicine the internal goods of healing and benevolence and the external good of financial compensation. For instance, hospital-based physicians know that their professional responsibility is to implement excellent diagnostic and therapeutic strategies so that a hospitalized patient recovers as quickly as possible and disease-related suffering as well as the risk of hospital-associated complications are thereby minimized. However, they are also aware that by limiting the length of a patient's stay in the hospital (i.e., by discharging a patient from the hospital sooner rather than later), more revenue will be received by the hospital due to the nature of diagnosis-associated payment mechanisms. In such a context, how do physicians stay focused on the health-centered needs of patients when they are also aware of the finance-centered needs of hospitals? Similarly, clinic-based physicians are aware of their professional obligations to promote health and minimize burdens for their patients. But they are also aware that under fee-for-service reimbursement mechanisms, more revenue comes from more return visits to the clinic, since clinic visits are billable. By contrast, follow-up provided by telephone or email communications may be medically appropriate and very convenient for patients, but they may not be compensated. How do physicians stay patient-centered in their

[24] Ibid., 191.

practice strategies in the midst of such financial incentives? These examples illustrate how real and relevant the distinction between internal and external goods can be.

The distinction between internal and external goods reminds us that tensions can arise whenever internal and external goods are pursued in tandem, which – MacIntyre reminds us – they always are. Institutions like hospitals are necessarily concerned with external goods. In the course of sustaining the *practice* of medicine, hospitals acquire, organize, and distribute external goods such as money, power, and status. These external goods pose challenges for a practice, but they are also necessary as the practical means by which practices are sustained over time.[25] The interrelationship of practices and institutions is intimate and tense:

> Indeed so intimate is the relationship of practices to institutions – and consequently of the goods external to the goods internal to the practices in question – that institutions and practices characteristically form a single causal order in which the ideals and the creativity of the practice are always vulnerable to the acquisitiveness of the institution, in which the cooperative care for common goods of the practice is always vulnerable to the competitiveness of the institution. In this context the essential function of the virtues is clear. Without them, without justice, courage and truthfulness, practices could not resist the corrupting power of institutions.[26]

The contrast MacIntyre draws warns us against the risk of confusing practices, and their internal goods, with institutions, and their external goods. This is a warning we should hear. But he presents the contrast so starkly that he runs the risk of implying that institutions are so focused on external goods that they cannot also be devoted to the internal goods of the practices they sponsor and sustain. We should therefore qualify MacIntyre's assessment by recognizing that institutions can be, if their leaders and members choose, genuinely devoted to the internal goods of the practices they sustain, even while they are also busy pursuing goods external to those practices. Good institutions, we might say, are those that place the purpose of a practice at the heart of their mission and allow that purpose to pervade and guide the entire organization and its activities. At their best, good institutions organize human endeavor in ways that promote valuable ends. They do so by setting expectations, maintaining standards, and creating structures and procedures that not only help achieve those ends but also support the moral values and integrity of

[25] Ibid., 194.
[26] Ibid.

individual professionals. It would be mistaken to invoke MacIntyre's account if to do so were to suggest that institutions are fundamentally opportunistic – exploiting practices for ulterior ends rather than supporting practices in their pursuit of internal goods. In short, we can qualify MacIntyre by suggesting that *good* institutions are *necessary for and supportive of* practices, even as we register his warning that challenges inevitably arise when external and internal goods are in tension.

Another illustration of the tension that can arise between the internal goods of medical practice and external goods related to financial gain can be seen in the conflicts of interest that exist when physicians are involved in financial relationships with pharmaceutical, device, or biotechnology companies, whether through compensation for services, royalties, or ownership interests.[27] Concerted attention to these conflicts has come from the federal government, state governments, professional organizations, medical schools, and hospitals. Concern arises from the conviction that patients' interests may be compromised if the actions of physicians are influenced by patient-centered interests *and* finance-centered interests. The definition of a conflict of interest as "a set of circumstances that creates a risk that professional judgment or actions regarding a primary interest will be unduly influenced by a secondary interest"[28] captures the contrast between an internal good (primary interest) and an external good (secondary interest) and makes it clear why the former must be prioritized over the latter. In recent years, health care institutions have had the opportunity to promote the *practice* of medicine by implementing structural changes to mitigate the extent to which physicians' financial conflicts are likely to undermine the interests of patients. This can be seen in the implementation of conflict-of-interest policies designed to protect the interests of patients against the possibly biasing influence of financial relationships with companies that physicians may choose to have. The emergence of such policies has been encouraged by societal and governmental pressures, but they have also been framed by ethical principles and driven by a concern to protect and cultivate a high standard of professional integrity.[29]

[27] Association of American Medical Colleges, *In the interest of patients: recommendations for physician financial relationships and clinical decision making* (Washington, DC, 2010), 10.

[28] Institute of Medicine, *Conflict of interest in medical research, education, and practice* (Washington, DC: National Academies Press, 2009), 46.

[29] D. J. Rothman and S. C. Chimonas, "New developments in managing physician–industry relationships," *JAMA* 300 (2008): 1067–69.

The preceding discussion has emphasized the goods and goals that define the practice of medicine, whether internally derived or externally imposed. Goals that are internally derived will inevitably also be influenced by society, since communities and governments have a legitimate interest in helping determine the nature and prioritization of medicine's goals. But in the process of this determination, the medical profession should be ready to articulate and defend its best understanding of the goods internal to medical practice in order to avoid the possibility of reducing medicine to a set of skills and techniques to be applied for whatever external purposes may be of interest to individuals, institutions, or society at a given point in time. MacIntyre's account of a practice indicates how the internal goods of the medical profession, and of institutions like hospitals, are essential if health care professionals are to function within and as part of a moral community. This function is characterized not simply by cooperation, but by virtues aligned with the internal goods of a practice that empower professionals to fulfill their purpose and, if need be, withstand externally imposed goals that contradict their purpose.

With this background of medicine as a practice defined by internally derived goods and goals in view, I turn now to clinical decision making in order to consider some of its morally challenging features and the need for an ethics of virtue capable of responding to these features with an approach to clinical reasoning based on goals of care.

IV. INSEPARABILITY OF CLINICAL DECISIONS AND ETHICAL VALUES

Because of the inherent moral value and physical embodiment of human beings, patients and physicians inhabit a world in which ethics and science are inseparable. As members of the human community, all patients are endowed with dignity that compels a fundamental respect for their needs and interests. A patient's dignity and a physician's promise to be a practitioner of healing combine to make the interaction between a patient and a physician an inherently moral encounter. The patient's value as a person obligates the physician to act in the patient's interests, as a fiduciary, implying that actions taken by a physician may be right or wrong, good or bad, to the extent that the moral requirements of the patient–physician encounter are, or are not, met. For these reasons medicine is a moral enterprise based on a covenant of trust.[30] In addition to its

[30] Ralph Crawshaw et al., "Patient–physician covenant," *JAMA* 273 (1995): 1553.

moral dimension, the practice of medicine reflects biological and technical realities understood through the methods of biomedical science. Decision making between patients and physicians therefore has a dual grounding in the values derived from ethics and the knowledge gained by science. Within this duality we see that science and technology show us what we *can* do in medicine and that ethics directs us to what we *should* do.

A review of codes of medical ethics, such as the *Code of Medical Ethics* of the American Medical Association and the *Ethics Manual* of the American College of Physicians, makes the ramifications of the relationship between ethics and science in medicine all too apparent. These documents represent normative responses to a wide range of ethical challenges in clinical practice, and the number of commonplace areas in which physicians may fail to live up to their profession's ethical standards is sobering. Because so many of these areas directly affect patients, physicians bear an enormous responsibility to act consistently in ways that respect patients and their interests. The significance of this responsibility explains why trust is essential when a patient is considering whether to follow a physician's recommendation.

To probe the interdependent relationship between ethics and science in clinical medicine, we might consider whether it could ever be seen as acceptable for a physician or surgeon to have great scientific and technical skill but be lacking in certain ethical values or commitments. One might imagine, for instance, a technically superior cardiologist whose primary motivation is to achieve financial success and for whom successful patient outcomes are first and foremost a means to personal financial gain. Might a patient be better off with a less superior cardiologist, but one who is primarily motivated by patients' needs and interests?

Albert Jonsen engages this question in an essay probing the nature of the therapeutic relationship. He concludes that we should not acquiesce to the suggestion that medical practice may be acceptable when technical competence is present but ethical uprightness is not.[31] He reaches this conclusion after exploring the "moral archeology" of medicine. There is, he maintains, an inherent tension arising from the profession's dual origins in Greek and medieval (Christian) medicine – the former justifying professional self-interest, the latter calling for professional altruism. In explaining his assessment, he analyzes two of the fundamental components of medical practice, diagnosis and therapy, and notes that each

[31] Albert R. Jonsen, "The therapeutic relationship: is moral conduct a necessary condition?" in *The clinical encounter*, ed. Shelp, 267–87.

component has a moral dimension that corresponds to a necessary virtue: diagnosis requires honesty (to pursue and communicate the truth), and therapy requires courage (to provide treatment that will or may cause suffering). Jonsen argues that the goals of diagnosis and therapy cannot be achieved in the absence of the corresponding virtues of honesty and courage. We could add to Jonsen's analysis by noting other ways in which these two virtues are of immediate relevance to medical practice, such as the courage to be honest after a medical error has been made. By pointing to the necessary association between skills and virtues in medicine, Jonsen helps us see how interdependent medicine and ethics are and how implausible it would be to suggest that brilliant technical skill (e.g., the "good hands" of a gifted surgeon) can ever be valuable enough to compensate for serious deficiencies in moral character.

Mark Siegler provides another perspective on the fundamentally ethical nature of medical practice by stressing the role played by the physician's moral beliefs and values in the patient–physician relationship.[32] When a patient comes to a physician, the encounter may or may not lead to what Siegler calls a doctor–patient accommodation, because the establishment of a medical relationship depends in large part on the physician's beliefs about what constitutes a medical problem. These beliefs are derived not only from a physician's biomedical knowledge, but also from the values that determine a physician's "standards of conscientious behavior."[33] These values may be shared within the profession or be individualized to the physician,[34] and they contribute to the multidimensional assessment by which physicians decide if a patient's problem is to be treated as a *medical* problem. Physicians, according to Siegler, "have the professional and personal responsibility, based on their training, expertise, and values, and modified by the existence of political, economic, and scientific boundaries to medicine, to weigh patient requests and to determine if they are to be managed, at least by *this* physician, as medical problems."[35]

The relationship between ethical values and scientific knowledge can also be seen in decision making shared by patients and physicians when the subjectivity of a specific patient's preferences is juxtaposed to the objectivity of the physician's professional understanding of the patient's good. Dan Brock explores this juxtaposition through what he calls the

[32] Mark Siegler, "The doctor–patient encounter and its relationship to theories of health and disease," in *Concepts of health and disease*, ed. Caplan et al., 627–44.

[33] Ibid., 641.

[34] Ibid., 642.

[35] Ibid., 643.

objective–subjective continuum, in which a patient's subjective values and preferences may at times conflict with that patient's objective good (which may be biological, physical, mental, or social).[36] This objective–subjective contrast explains how a physician may at times be justified in countering a patient's expressed preferences if the physician is serving as an advocate for that patient's objective good. Brock recognizes, of course, that the self-determination of a competent patient must ultimately decide the course of action taken, since freedom – at least the freedom to be left alone – is an even more fundamental aspect of a patient's objective good. The legitimacy of physician advocacy for a patient's objective good reflects the fact that medical practice is value-laden and value-directed – that is, it assumes that medical practice is supposed to pursue certain goods, such as health, comfort, and the prevention of disease. These values allow physicians, and indeed require them, to be professing promoters of goods rather than value-neutral providers of biomedical facts apart from their relevance to these goods. It is this basic orientation to the goods of health care, when grounded in respect for human dignity and accompanied by ethical values expected of medical professionals (such as truthfulness, confidentiality, and altruism), that makes medical practice the moral enterprise it needs to be.

V. UNIQUENESS OF CLINICAL CIRCUMSTANCES

The promotion of goods such as health, comfort, and many forms of disease prevention ultimately occurs at the level of particular persons, and this means that the practice of clinical medicine always entails a certain uniqueness that arises from the particularity of each encounter between an individual patient and an individual physician. As a result, clinical decision making always depends on the features of a specific person, a specific condition or disease and its specific manifestations, and a specific set of circumstances that surround the individual involved. The practice of medicine always unfolds as an individualized event, and the advent of "personalized" or "individualized" medicine in the era of genomic science has only heightened our awareness of how individualized diseases and their treatments can be. The individualized nature of health care arises not only in response to person-specific differences in the expression or

[36] Dan W. Brock, "Facts and values in the physician–patient relationship," in *Ethics, trust, and the professions: philosophical and cultural aspects*, ed. E. D. Pellegrino, R. M. Veatch, and J. P. Langan (Washington, DC: Georgetown University Press, 1991), 113–30.

impact a disease or condition may have (arising from needs that may be genetic, physiological, psychological, sociological, or economical in origin),[37] but also as part of a patient-centered approach to care that tailors decision making to the unique preferences of each patient. Moreover, if we also include physicians and their particularity in our considerations, we can see the uniqueness of each clinical encounter as arising from at least two persons, each bringing to the encounter his or her own constellation of variables (such as personality, character, temperament, values, beliefs, and motivations)[38] that will in large measure determine how the patient–physician interaction proceeds. The dependence of this interaction on the particularity of the persons involved should never be underestimated.

The clinical encounter is a meeting between a person in need, the patient, and a person professing a readiness to meet that need, the physician. (By focusing on the clinical encounter as it pertains to *physicians,* I do not mean to deny the obvious fact that clinical encounters routinely include other health care professionals, who may work independently or with physicians in teams.) Ideally, the responsibility for decisions aimed at addressing the need is shared by the patient and the physician. Through dialogue, relevant information is disclosed by both parties, leading to a shared understanding of the patient's beliefs, concerns, and goals, as well as the physician's assessment of the problem and its possible causes and remedies. A physician gathers information from the patient's current and previous experiences (history of the present illness and past medical history), from an evaluation of the patient's body (physical examination), and from technological investigations of the patient's body or bodily substances (laboratory and radiographic testing). Depending on the interpretation of this information, the patient may be advised to modify behaviors, take medications, or undergo a procedure or surgery. The ease and speed with which this sequence of events is repeated by physicians every day should not lessen our appreciation for its profound dependence on the particularity of the persons involved. The particularity of this encounter will determine what information is provided and how it is communicated (by patient and physician), what data are collected and how they are interpreted, and what recommendations are made and how advice is followed. It is for such reasons that

[37] Engelhardt, "The concepts of health and disease," 37.

[38] Siegler, "The doctor–patient encounter and its relationship to theories of health and disease," 638.

"standardized" care is hard to achieve – even when there is consensus among professionals regarding best practices.

Thankfully, there is much professional consensus covering large amounts of medical practice, with the result that many physicians and patients approach many medical problems in a relatively uniform fashion. For example, the medical approach to the assessment of chest pain is sufficiently grounded in clinical experience and evidence, and sufficiently emphasized in clinical training, that when a patient complains of pain in the region of the chest, there will predictably follow a series of evaluative steps, usually prompt, guided by a concern for possibly life-threatening diagnoses – such as a heart attack, a blood clot in the lungs, or a disruption of the major artery in the chest (the aorta). But it is equally true that even in the evaluation of a complaint as routinely encountered as chest pain, there will still be variability in the process of evaluation and decision making. Variability will arise from the way the pain is communicated by the patient and interpreted by the physician, the physician's level of experience and degree of attention, the patient's trust in the physician's judgment, the extent of medical information the physician provides, and the circumstances surrounding the patient and physician (such as time of day or night, presence and support of family members, cost of care, level of inconvenience, pressures of time, and presence of competing responsibilities). These and other aspects illustrate how each patient–physician encounter is contingent on the unique features of the persons involved and their circumstances. What might in a textbook be described as a standardized protocol of decision making under the rubric "Evaluation and Treatment of Chest Pain" will often turn out in real life to be a process that is abbreviated, improvised, or circuitous. Patients and physicians manifest particularity, and the processes and outcomes of many of their encounters are unpredictable to the extent that "standard" approaches to care may be modified or set aside because of the particularities that drive decision making.

In light of the uniqueness of each patient–physician encounter, the inseparability of clinical decisions and ethical values is all the more significant. So much about decision making depends on a particular physician's ability to listen, inquire, interpret, assess, advise, and gain trust. Much also depends on a physician's beliefs about the merits and sincerity of a patient's concerns, as well as a physician's responsiveness to a patient's dignity and vulnerability. Such characteristics of physicians should be expected to play significant and potentially decisive roles in how they make decisions with patients. Their influence can become highly evident when physicians care for patients they perceive as "difficult," whether because of a diagnosis (e.g., terminal illness, dementia, substance abuse, or HIV infection), socioeconomic status, linguistic or cultural differences, or uncooperative or demanding behaviors. In such circumstances, the strength of a professional's motivation is tested, and a physician's particular virtues will determine how hard and patiently she will work to promote the best interests of a patient.

Another dimension of the uniqueness of the patient–physician encounter involves the particular beliefs and values each person brings to his or her assessment of issues that are explicitly ethical. Whether it is a matter of informed consent, confidentiality, perinatal care, end-of-life care, or surrogate decision making – different beliefs and values will lead to different interpretations or assignments of priority when competing values or interests are hard to reconcile. A physician's response to an ethical challenge or dilemma will depend on her moral beliefs and values and how these are integrated into her assessments and recommendations.

The impact of a physician's particular moral beliefs and values is also manifested in the way she perceives the circumstances that occasion a challenging ethical situation. There is a long moral tradition that reminds us that ethical decision making must to a large extent be a case-by-case endeavor, as opposed to a strictly rule-based process. Aristotle, for instance, said that it is not possible to lay down in advance specific moral rules for action, since circumstances will always vary and should be allowed to guide ethical decision making.[39] Thomas Aquinas likewise recognized the dependence of individual cases on their particular circumstances, though he also thought that certain kinds of actions, such as killing innocent people, are always wrong.[40] Following both Aristotle and Aquinas, Josef Pieper maintained that ethical approaches should not attempt to calculate moral action in advance and in the abstract, but instead should use prudence to respond appropriately to the actual circumstances of a given case.[41] A physician's responsiveness to the concrete details of a unique set of circumstances will inevitably depend on what she perceives those details to be, which in turn will depend on what moral beliefs and values she brings to the interrelated processes of perception and evaluation.

39 David Bostock, *Aristotle's ethics* (Oxford: Oxford University Press, 2000), 5.
40 Brian Davies, *The thought of Thomas Aquinas* (Oxford: Clarendon Press, 1993), 237–39.
41 Josef Pieper, *The four cardinal virtues* (Notre Dame, IN: University of Notre Dame Press, 1966), 27–28.

VI. GOALS OF CARE FOR GOAL-DIRECTED DECISION MAKING IN MEDICINE

This chapter describes the moral character of medicine in terms of its internal goods, ethical values, particularity, and goals. To appreciate why goals are so central to ethical decision making in medicine, we need to explore their significance further. To begin, there are two tendencies in contemporary medical practice that make goals particularly meaningful for decision making shared by patients and physicians. First, there is a common tendency to expect patients to know and be able to communicate their treatment preferences, often without the benefit of dialogue with physicians that would allow them to explain and explore the reasons for those preferences. Second, there is a common tendency to let possible actions (e.g., proposed tests or treatments) trigger and thereby frame decision making, rather than to allow broader purposes (goals) to guide possible actions. The first tendency is fueled by the understandably heavy emphasis placed on respect for patient autonomy in contemporary medical practice, especially when it is manifested by soliciting patients' choices about specific treatments without necessarily probing the reasons for those treatments. The second tendency is arguably driven by the heavy emphasis on interventional technologies in medical practice that encourage health professionals toward an almost automatic focus on what *can* be done rather than on what *should* be done, leaving the latter consideration mainly to the dictates of patient choice – and in turn suggesting that these two tendencies have the potential to be mutually reinforcing.

In contrast to an approach to decision making that consists of options described by physicians and choices articulated by patients, goal-oriented decision making encourages patients to view their options against the backdrop of their guiding beliefs and values. Goal-based decision making does not deny the importance of patient preference; rather, it emphasizes the need to ensure that patient preferences are based on beliefs and values that are consistent with their broader and deeper purposes and thereby provide a more meaningful and enduring context for making choices. The more a decision focuses on medical interventions rather than on goals, the more likely it is that the availability of an intervention will suggest its advisability.

As an illustration of the need for goal-oriented decision making, consider discussions physicians have with hospitalized patients or their families about cardiopulmonary resuscitation (CPR) in the event of a cardiac or pulmonary arrest. Experience suggests that these discussions are usually framed in terms of treatment preferences, focusing intensely on whether or not a specific intervention (CPR) should be performed in case of a specific event (cardiac or pulmonary arrest). By concentrating narrowly on the intervention, such discussions tend to be dislocated from the larger context of meaning that goals can provide. If a physician can first clarify with a patient or family what goals are most important (e.g., curing a disease, prolonging life, restoring function, or being comfortable), then the benefits and burdens of CPR can be assessed in light of those goals.[42]

To appreciate the significance of goals in medical decision making is to see that when medicine is guided by goals it is a teleological process – that is, a process oriented toward ends, the achievement of which constitutes medicine's success. When an action is directed toward a goal (i.e., a good and desirable objective or thing), the action's orientation to that goal is part of the action's goodness. Within a teleological account like this, whether an action is good or bad depends on whether it is or is not oriented to a good goal – as well as on the action's intrinsic quality and surrounding circumstances.[43] In a general sense, it is right to say, simply, that insofar as a person has a reason for action, that action is oriented to a goal.[44] In contrasting goal-oriented decisions with intervention-oriented decisions, I do not intend to suggest that intervention-oriented actions are completely lacking with respect to goals. At some level, every decision in medicine has a goal to the extent that it has a reason behind it. But I believe it is appropriate to suggest that some decisions in medicine are so focused on interventions that the reasons for making them reflect what is available, convenient, or routine rather than what is advisable in light of the patient's particular beliefs and values. Intervention-focused decision making tends to concentrate on the most direct means of addressing the most immediate aspects of a medical problem, without first taking into consideration the patient's broader and more enduring goals. Intervention-focused decision making therefore has a quality of expediency, typically driven by a felt need to take action, to "do something." By contrast, goal-directed decision making strives to reflect patients' beliefs and values by identifying their goals of care and then assessing the merits

[42] T. G. Gehlbach et al., "Code status orders and goals of care in the medical intensive care unit," *Chest* 139 (2011): 802–809.

[43] Thomas Aquinas, *Summa theologica: a concise translation*, trans. Timothy McDermott (Westminster, MD: Christian Classics, 1989), 196–97.

[44] Ralph McInerny, "Ethics," in *Aquinas*, ed. Norman Kretzmann and Eleonore Stump (Cambridge: Cambridge University Press, 1993), 198.

of possible interventions in light of those goals. Goal-directed decision making tries to pause long enough to establish a context of meaning and purpose that can guide action.

The contrast between interventions and goals is of great practical relevance in clinical medicine, especially when ethical questions arise. In cases of ethical uncertainty or disagreement, discussions between patients and professionals tend too often to revolve around the question of whether a specific intervention should be initiated, continued, or discontinued. The focus on interventions is natural and necessary for clinicians, given their intervention-centered training, the host of treatments medicine has to offer, the potential for interventions to change the course of disease for the patient's benefit, and the urgent and emergent conditions that demand prompt decisions in order to administer rapid remedies. The common risk, however, is that a physician may devote so much attention to discussing an intervention that the broader context and purpose of a patient's care may be neglected or obscured. The risk of losing sight of the larger landscape of a patient's condition and health-related priorities by focusing too narrowly on interventions indicates why goals of care are so important. Goals provide a frame of reference that orients clinical decision making toward what is believed to be most worth pursuing. As a destination orients a traveler, so goals direct medical decision making. In the absence of goals, interventional choices are more likely to be isolated and reactionary rather than integrated and proactive.

Earlier in this chapter I mentioned a group of international scholars convened by the Hastings Center to identify goals that should guide the practice of medicine. The work of this group was motivated in part by eight concerns about the practice of medicine and characteristics of society: (1) scientific and technological developments; (2) the curative bias of medicine; (3) the aging of the population; (4) free-market forces and growing public demands; (5) cultural pressures; (6) society's tendency to "medicalize" aspects of human life not traditionally under the domain of medicine; (7) interest in the enhancement of human abilities; and (8) the consequences of not having appropriate goals (economic unsustainability, clinical confusion, social frustration, and incoherent directions).[45]

These scholars are not the first to have drawn attention to the complex and widespread forces that bear upon the practice of medicine. Leon Kass, for instance, has expressed such concerns, finding it ironic "that

[45] Hanson and Callahan, *The goals of medicine*, 7–13.

medicine's great technical power should arrive in tandem with great confusion about the standards and goals for guiding its use."[46] Kass argues not only that medicine is troubled by uncertainty about its goals, but also that there are false goals to be avoided, such as the satisfaction of pleasure or desire, behavior modification, the alteration of human nature, and the attempt to prevent death as if it were something that did not have to be accepted.[47] Both Kass and the Hastings Center scholars note society's tendency to engage the broad challenges of medicine by managing and modifying the *means* employed by medicine rather than addressing its *ends.* This tendency results in intense technical discussions that obscure questions about the purpose of medicine,[48] and thus medicine ends up being treated merely as a set of powerful means and the physician merely as a technician of the body.[49] These concerns help explain why the task of clarifying the goals of medicine is such a vital challenge.

The Hastings Center group took up that challenge and identified four goals of medicine:

1. the prevention of disease and injury and the promotion and maintenance of health;
2. the relief of pain and suffering caused by maladies;
3. the care and cure of those with a malady and the care of those who cannot be cured; and
4. the avoidance of premature death and the pursuit of a peaceful death.[50]

They were unwilling to give any of these goals priority over the others, and they acknowledged that the first goal is not only for medicine but also for society, since its achievement requires collaboration with organizations and resources beyond the medical profession. The authors also addressed the question of the universal validity of these goals, concluding they should be accepted as universally valid given the shared reality of human nature and the common human experiences of sickness, pain, suffering, accident, injury, and dependence on others for care.[51] The authors make a compelling case, and I believe their four goals constitute a concise articulation of the core purposes that continue to guide and

46 Kass, "Regarding the end of medicine and the pursuit of health," 4.
47 Ibid., 5–7.
48 Hanson and Callahan, *The goals of medicine*, 4.
49 Kass, "Regarding the end of medicine and the pursuit of health," 4.
50 Hanson and Callahan, *The goals of medicine*, 21–30.
51 Ibid., 14–15.

justify the practice of medicine. This is not to deny room for debate about the exact number, terminology, or boundaries of such goals, but it is to claim that grounds for their validity should be available on the basis of their generality as well as widespread convictions about medicine and ethics that support these four goals.

In addition to this list of goals that express the most overarching purposes of medicine and public health, it is important to consider how goals are formulated in the context of clinical care for individual patients, which we may refer to as *goals of care*. Recent efforts have helped clarify how goals of care can be specified in clinically relevant terms that can facilitate decision making shared by patients and clinicians.[52] Such work has identified seven goals of care that can be discussed with patients to clarify the underlying reasons for patients' treatment preferences and then provide orientation for their implementation:

1. to cure a patient;
2. to help a patient live longer;
3. to improve or maintain a patient's function/quality of life/independence;
4. to help a patient be comfortable;
5. to help a patient achieve his or her life goals;
6. to provide support for a patient's family/caregivers; and
7. to clarify a patient's diagnosis or prognosis.

Discussing and prioritizing these goals help patients and physicians articulate goal-oriented assessments and preferences that can guide decision making and increase the likelihood that treatment decisions will harmonize with patients' beliefs and values, as well as with the reality of their medical conditions.

As a conceptual framework for communication and decision making, goals of care are relevant to all of clinical medicine, even if in some domains, like end-of-life care or discussions about cardiopulmonary resuscitation,[53] their pertinence is especially clear. This general relevance derives from the relationship between goals and interventions in clinical

[52] Lauris C. Kaldjian et al., "Goals of care toward the end of life: a structured literature review," *American Journal of Hospice and Palliative Medicine* 25 (2009): 501–11; T. H. Haberle et al., "Goals of care among hospitalized patients: a validation study," *American Journal of Hospice and Palliative Medicine* 28 (2010): 335–41.

[53] Lauris C. Kaldjian et al., "Code status discussions and goals of care among hospitalized adults," *Journal of Medical Ethics* 35 (2009): 338–42; Gehlbach et al., "Code status orders and goals of care in the medical intensive care unit."

medicine, as seen by the relationship between three basic elements in the patient–physician encounter: what is understood (diagnosis, prognosis), what is being considered (intervention), and what is intended (goals of care). In order for an intervention to be properly helpful, it has to have a proper relation to the patient's condition and to the patient's goals of care, and the propriety of that relation is gauged by the likelihood that an intervention (like a transporting vehicle, to use the analogy of travel) will move the patient toward that goal of care. The reasonableness of an intervention will depend on the degree of coherence between the patient's condition, the intervention, and goals of care; and this degree is determined not only by the patient's assessment of the perceived benefits and risks of an intervention, but also by a medically informed prediction based on all available data. Once clarified, goals of care allow clinicians, patients, and families to discuss whether an intervention is likely to be a reasonable means to a particular end. Ideally, decisions about interventions should therefore emerge from, rather than lead to, discussions about goals of care. To use the analogy of travel again, a destination should guide, not follow, the choice and route of transportation.

As important as they are, goals of care are not without challenges. The more general a goal is, the more interpretation it will require and the more uncertainty its meaning will have. When a patient has more than one important goal – which is commonly the case – there is the possibility of tension between goals that may require prioritizing. For example, a patient with a curable illness facing a highly burdensome treatment may decide to place the goal of cure above the goal of comfort; or a patient dying from painful terminal cancer may decide to place the goal of consciousness (to preserve the ability to communicate with family members) above the goal of comfort (treatments for which might be accompanied by the side effect of sedation). Diagnostic and prognostic clarity also has an impact on goals. The more certain the diagnosis and prognosis, the easier it is to determine which goals of care are realistic based on the features of a particular disease with its known trajectory, known treatments, and known treatment-related burdens. It is difficult to decide on appropriate goals when diagnoses and prognoses are uncertain. This is why clarifying the diagnosis or prognosis is sometimes the most pressing goal of care. When diagnostic or prognostic uncertainties exist, time-limited treatment trials may be needed to assess the results of empiric ("best educated guess") interventions. Goals also shift over time, as biological realities change during the course of illness and as personal preferences adjust to those changing realities. One of the greatest skills physicians need is the ability to help patients make the transition from one set of goals to another, through anticipation of disease trajectories, attention to unfolding medical facts, and ongoing dialogue.

At times there may be deep disagreements among patients, family members, physicians, or other health professionals regarding the appropriateness or priority of a given goal of care. For example, a family may prefer that a patient's life be prolonged by intensive life-supporting means, while a physician may believe that continued life support will not likely prolong life by more than a few days or weeks but will prolong suffering and consume professional time and other resources. Such disagreements remind us that the choice of goals in a given case will always depend on the guiding beliefs and values of the persons involved. Interventions should be oriented by goals, and goals should be informed by biomedical realities. But the *choice* of goals will also be shaped by beliefs and values related to fundamental concerns, such as the value of prolonging an individual human life for a limited time, the acceptability of suffering, the significance attributed to specific outcome probabilities, and the costs of treatment. When disagreements arise, the rationale for different goals may have to be explained and negotiated in the hope that dialogue will lead to consensus or that intractable differences can somehow be accommodated. When conflicts persist, articulating goals may have the benefit of clarifying the nature of the disagreement so that all involved may understand whether the dispute is about competing goals or about competing means to achieve a shared goal. And even when disagreements over goals resist the most compassionate and respectful attempts at resolution, careful discussions may help identify deeply held beliefs and values that underlie goal preferences, which may increase mutual understanding and thereby make disagreement less disturbing and disruptive.

Dialogues with patients about goals of care require an unusual set of communication skills on the part of the clinician. Careful consideration must be given to (1) how to initiate the discussion; (2) how to explain complex medical details in understandable language; (3) how to make space for and respond to questions, listen to emotional responses, and "read" the patient's readiness to make decisions; (4) how to help patients identify and apply their guiding ethical, spiritual, or religious beliefs and values; (5) how to lay out an appropriate range of treatment alternatives while also making (when appropriate) specific recommendations; (6) how to sustain hope in the midst of disappointing and fearful realities as medical crises arise and diseases progress; and (7) how to orchestrate transitions in goals of care with candor and compassion over the course of a progressive illness. This last skill is perhaps the greatest challenge, as it requires great sensitivity to the changing medical conditions and emotional and spiritual needs of the patient in order to guide stepwise transitions that move, in time, from the "full court press" of curative therapy to the "comfort measures only" of palliation.

VII. ADDITIONAL DIMENSIONS OF DECISION MAKING: PROBABILITIES, SUFFERING, AND COST

It would be misleading to discuss goals of care without acknowledging two other core dimensions of decision making that are essential for facilitating good decisions about interventional options. The first of these pertains to probabilities. Patients and physicians need to discuss the outcome probabilities (both positive and negative) associated with interventional options, even though there are many challenges to communicating and understanding probabilistic information. Sometimes the statistical likelihood of achieving a desired goal (or suffering a complication) from a given intervention may turn out to be a decisive factor in deciding whether or not to pursue that goal. Patients' diverse assessments of the personal significance of different probabilities make the discussion of probabilities essential in every patient's case. Physicians cannot know in advance of discussion what probabilities a given patient will interpret as sufficiently high or low to affect decision making.

The other additional dimension of decision making pertains to a patient's willingness to endure suffering due to the physical and emotional burdens that medical treatment often entails. A patient may understand his diagnosis and prognosis, identify his goals of care, and accept a given probability of achieving those goals by means of a specific intervention. Yet there is still the question of how much he is willing to go through in order to achieve his goals under the given conditions. Some interventions may have high probabilities of success, yet they can impose such heavy physical or emotional burdens that patients may decline to undergo them. The dimension of suffering will always be a part of decision making when medical treatment entails significant burdens that can be anticipated and need to be weighed in the balance.

There is one other dimension of decision making that may or may not be considered a direct professional concern for the process of decision making shared by individual patients and physicians, and this is the dimension of financial cost. Beyond goals, probabilities, and suffering, if financial resources are scarce or unavailable, treatment may be economically inadvisable or practically impossible. Costs raise vexing questions about fairness and the need for distributive justice in the provision of health services based on medical need, whether that distribution is within communities, countries, or across the globe. The dimension of cost in a given clinical situation may be direct or indirect, explicit or implicit, but it is always there. The questions for the purpose of this discussion are whether and how individual physicians should incorporate cost considerations into shared decision making with individual patients – and this is a controversial issue.

Some would argue that physicians have a dual responsibility to care for individual patients, one at a time, while simultaneously fulfilling an obligation to benefit society by controlling health care costs through the so-called bedside rationing of health care.[54] Those opposed to this view believe that the obligation to control costs should not fall on individual physicians caring for patients; they emphasize the need to preserve trust between patients and physicians and to avoid the risk of discrimination through unjust allocation of health care resources.[55] Some who share concerns about excessive or unsustainable health care costs, but disagree that physicians ought to have a direct, bedside role in controlling those costs through rationing, prefer to place the burden of cost control on administrators and governments so physicians can serve as unconflicted advocates for their patients even as they are obliged to follow the cost-containing directives authorized at higher organizational levels within a health care system.[56]

Arguments against the direct rationing of health services by physicians take seriously the *role-fidelity* that guards a physician's fiduciary responsibility to serve as an advocate for his patients, whenever possible, one at a time. Admittedly, in situations involving mass casualties or in resource-constrained settings like the intensive care unit,[57] an individual physician may have to serve as the advocate for multiple patients simultaneously through triage decisions that weigh the benefits of treating individual

[54] Peter A. Ubell, "Physicians, thou shalt ration: the necessary role of bedside rationing in controlling healthcare costs," *Healthcare Papers* 2 (2001): 10–21.

[55] Arthur Schafer, "Bedside rationing by physicians: the case against," *Healthcare Papers* 2 (2001): 45–52.

[56] Sigurd Lauridsen, "Administrative gatekeeping: a third way between unrestricted patient advocacy and bedside rationing," *Bioethics* 23 (2009): 311–20.

[57] Michael J. Young et al., "Rationing in the intensive care unit: to disclose or disguise?" *Critical Care Medicine* 40 (2012): 261–66.

patients against each other and, thereby, ration care. But apart from such uniquely challenging settings where immediate access to needed resources is limited, the argument against direct rationing by physicians assumes that cost-controlling strategies in health care should respect a division of labor that separates administrative decisions about access to resources from clinical decisions about the need for those resources. This "division of labor" position holds that physicians should not attempt to serve simultaneously as advocates for the health of individual patients and as stewards for the economic health of society. It maintains that physicians should, generally speaking, be care providers, not resource allocators – even as it acknowledges that policy decisions based on economic constraints will necessarily limit what forms and amounts of medical care patients will be allowed to receive.

In recent years concerns about health care costs have increasingly led to professional recommendations promoting the physician's dual responsibility to provide medical care that both meets the needs of individual patients and controls the overall costs of care to society. Even though these recommendations stress the need to avoid wasteful or unnecessarily expensive care rather than to limit or ration care, they represent a shift away from a *primary* focus on the *patient–physician dyad* to what we might call a *patient–physician–population triad*. This can be seen in recent positions taken by medical organizations, such as the American Medical Association, emphasizing that physicians have a professional responsibility of stewardship that obliges them to consider the cost of care when making medical decisions.[58] In some cases organizations stress the need for stewardship while also acknowledging the need for a division of labor. The American College of Physicians (ACP) holds that physicians have "an ethical responsibility to provide health care services that are necessary and effective and not to provide care that is ineffective, inappropriate, or harmful," but the ACP also states that "resource allocation decisions concerning use of limited health care resources must also be made at a policy level for the health care system."[59] To separate the policy challenge of resource allocation at the level of society from the challenge of medical decision making at the level of the individual patient, the ACP draws a helpful distinction between *rationing* medical treatments, whereby

[58] Kevin B. O'Reilly, "Doctors advised to consider costs in care choices," *American Medical News*, July 9, 2012.

[59] ACP, "How can our nation conserve and distribute health care resources effectively and efficiently?" (Philadelphia: American College of Physicians, 2011).

someone decides which scarce medical resources are provided and to whom, and *rational* medical decision making, in which "judicious choices are made among clinically effective alternatives."[60] The consequence of rationing is a denial of treatment; the purpose of rational decision making is to maximize value by choosing the most appropriate treatment option among alternatives with different costs and benefits. The ACP's interest in controlling the costs of care has resulted in a new program, the High Value, Cost Conscious Care initiative.[61] This initiative is designed to help physicians provide excellent care to their patients while also taking seriously the costs of intervention by avoiding the overuse and misuse of resources that do not improve outcomes and may cause harm.[62]

Given the need to improve the fair distribution of health care resources to all persons in need of medical care and to do so within society's economic limitations, we ought to support systems of care that encourage physicians to practice evidence-based, patient-centered, and cost-effective medicine. But we ought to do so without placing on physicians' shoulders a responsibility for controlling health care costs in ways that may decrease their commitment to advocating for individual patients as they increase their commitment to the "greater good" of society. Given the human limitations physicians face in their ability to distribute health care services without favoring some patients over others, it would not be morally realistic to expect them to shoulder the responsibility of micro-allocating resources fairly. We should not place more responsibility on the backs of physicians than they can bear. True to the spirit of a representative democracy and its rationale for the separation of powers, we should rely on a division of labor to ensure that individual patients have advocates in physicians and that populations have advocates in administrators and legislators. It can be noted in passing that the controversy over the physician's appropriate role in controlling health care costs nicely illustrates some of the key concerns of this chapter – the internal and external goods of medical practice, the inseparability of clinical decisions and ethical values, and the goals that should guide medical practice.

[60] Ibid.

[61] Cynthia D. Smith, "Teaching high-value, cost-conscious care to residents: the Alliance for Academic Internal Medicine–American College of Physicians curriculum," *Annals of Internal Medicine* 157 (2012): 284–86.

[62] Douglas K. Owens et al., "High-value, cost-conscious health care: concepts for clinicians to evaluate the benefits, harms, and costs of medical interventions," *Annals of Internal Medicine* 154 (2011): 174–80.

VIII. SUMMARY

Physicians and other health care professionals need the virtue of practical wisdom in order to respond well to the wide range of challenging decisions that caring for patients involves. Practical wisdom is directed toward ends or goals, so to understand what practical wisdom means in medicine, we must first understand what its goals should be. These goals arise from an understanding of the goods that medicine is supposed to pursue, goods that may be defined by values believed to be inherent in the nature of medical practice (the essentialist view), values determined by society (the socially constructed view), or values medical professionals impose on the practice of medicine (the professionally constructed view). Differences of opinion concerning what or who ought to determine the goals of medicine may also be accompanied by differences of interpretation about underlying concepts of health and disease. By attending to these differences, we are reminded of the diverse ways in which people may perceive medicine and its goals. In the midst of these actual or potential differences, it is important to maintain a view that includes an objective assessment of health and disease based on biomedical science, even as it encompasses the subjective ways in which health and disease are experienced and the diverse interpretations they receive from patients, societies, and cultures. Such a view is of great relevance to the patient–physician relationship, in which dialogues should engage the particular beliefs and needs of individual patients without denying the objective validity of the knowledge and skill that professionals gain from biomedical science and clinical experience.

To understand more fully the goods believed to be inherent in medical practice, it is helpful to consider MacIntyre's analysis of the relationship between virtues and the notion of a practice. On his account, internal goods (like healing and comforting in medicine) are a defining feature of a practice, recognized through participation in the practice and adoption of its rules and standards. The fulfillment of these goods is not merely the accomplishment of an individual professional, but a success for all professionals in that practice. Pursuit of the internal goods of the medical profession is essential to its function as a moral community. This function is characterized not simply by cooperation, but by a shared commitment to virtues that are aligned with the internal goods of a practice and that empower professionals to fulfill their goals together and, if need be, withstand externally imposed priorities that contradict those goals. Tensions between internal goods, such as healing and comforting, and external goods, such as money and prestige, can exist for an individual professional (e.g., when conflicts of interest arise) or between professionals and their institutions when goals come into conflict.

When we understand medicine as a moral practice defined primarily by its internal goods, we can appreciate how inextricably biomedical science is linked with ethics and how important it is to distinguish between the scientific-technical powers of medicine and the ends or goals that those powers are supposed to serve. The inseparability of science and ethics in medicine explains why a physician's ethical values cannot be separated from the scientifically informed interpretations and judgments that determine her clinical recommendations and the nature of her role in shared decision making with patients. That role depends on a physician's judgments about the proper scope of medical practice, on virtues such as honesty and courage, on managing the tension between self-interest and altruism, and on the moral beliefs and values that underlie a physician's decisions.

Decision making shared by a physician and patient is a unique process of engagement between one person in need and another professing to be ready to meet that need, both of whom come to the encounter with particular beliefs, values, and expectations that will together determine what the outcome of the encounter will be. The particularity of patients and physicians means that clinical and ethical decision making will always be an individualized process based on a range of patient and physician characteristics. When specifically ethical questions arise, these characteristics will include the moral beliefs and values that patients and physicians (and other involved parties) bring to the clinical encounter.

Decisions about medical interventions should emerge from discussions about goals of care. Goals provide a frame of reference for shared decision making that orients decisions about interventions toward a goal that is determined by a patient's guiding beliefs and values. In the absence of goals, choices about tests and treatments are likely to be isolated and reactionary rather than integrated and proactive. Common goals of care include (1) to cure a patient; (2) to help a patient live longer; (3) to improve or maintain a patient's function/quality of life/independence; (4) to help a patient be comfortable; (5) to help a patient achieve his or her life goals; (6) to provide support for a patient's family/caregivers; and (7) to clarify a patient's diagnosis or prognosis. Identifying which of these goals are most important helps guide decision making and increases the likelihood that treatment decisions will harmonize with patients' beliefs and values and with their medical conditions. When disagreements arise about goals of care, the rationale for specific goals may have to be explained to increase mutual understanding and work towards consensus. Articulating goals may also have the benefit of clarifying the nature of disagreements so that it becomes clear whether a dispute involves competing goals or competing means to achieve a shared goal. In addition to goals of care, shared decision making ought to incorporate two other dimensions: the probability of a given intervention's success and the amount of suffering, or burden, the intervention is anticipated to impose.

A further dimension to consider is financial cost, and this raises questions about whether and how individual physicians should incorporate cost considerations into shared decision making with individual patients. This is a controversial issue that entails, on one side, those who claim physicians have a stewardship responsibility to exercise so-called bedside rationing and, on the other, those who claim that any such attempts will diminish the trust between patients and physicians and create injustices due to discriminatory allocation decisions. Arguments against the direct rationing of health services by physicians emphasize the role-fidelity that guards a physician's fiduciary responsibility to serve as a patient advocate. Some who share concerns about excessive or unsustainable health care costs but disagree with bedside rationing would place the burden of cost control squarely on administrators and governments so physicians can serve as unconflicted advocates for their patients while also following cost-containing restrictions authorized at higher organizational levels within a health care system. This allows for a "division of labor" by which individual physicians advocate for individual patients, and administrators advocate for populations.

Professional recommendations promoting the physician's responsibility to provide medical care that meets the needs of individual patients *and* controls the costs of care to society are increasing. These recommendations represent a shift from a traditional focus on the patient–physician dyad to a patient–physician–population triad, and they stress the need to avoid wasteful or unnecessarily expensive care. Given the need to improve the fair distribution of health care resources in an economically constrained environment, physicians ought to practice evidence-based, patient-centered, and cost-effective medicine. But this does not mean we should place on physicians' shoulders a responsibility for controlling health care costs in ways that may decrease their advocacy for individual patients as they increase their commitment to the "greater good" of society. The debate about a physician's proper role in the control of health care costs illustrates key concerns in this chapter regarding the internal and external goods of medical practice, the inseparability of clinical decisions and ethical values, and the goals that should guide medical practice.

2

Virtue Ethics

I. DISTINCTIVE FEATURES OF VIRTUE ETHICS

A. Thinking, Doing, and Being

Virtue ethics provides a framework of meaning in which the virtue of practical wisdom can be defined, related to other virtues, and contrasted with other approaches to normative ethics such as those that rely primarily on principles or consequences. *Principle-based* (deontological) theories place the emphasis of morality on duties of obligation and emphasize the rightness or wrongness of certain kinds of *actions*, such as killing or lying. *Consequence-based* (consequentialist or utilitarian) theories place the emphasis on the overall *outcomes* of actions and the goodness or badness of those outcomes, such as the consequences of killing or lying. *Virtue-based* theories place the emphasis on persons and the fundamental importance of *what kind of people we are and want to be* (e.g., nonviolent or honest), directing our attention to *being*,[1] in contrast to thinking and doing. Virtue ethics assumes that how one thinks and acts depends on who one is, in a moral sense,[2] such that one's character determines one's choices.[3] Since as far back as Aristotle (384–322 B.C.E.), virtue ethics has brought to the fore concerns about traits of character, focusing primarily on what kind of person one ought to *be* rather than on – as with most modern ethical theories – what one ought to *do*.[4]

[1] William Frankena, *Ethics* (Englewood Cliffs, NJ: Prentice Hall, 1973), 63.

[2] Gilbert C. Meilaender, *The theory and practice of virtue* (Notre Dame, IN: University of Notre Dame Press, 1984), 5.

[3] Stanley Hauerwas, "Reconciling the practice of reason: casuistry in a Christian context," in *Moral theory and moral judgments in medical ethics*, ed. Baruch A. Brody (Dordrecht: Kluwer Academic, 1988), 137.

[4] Bostock, *Aristotle's ethics*: 51.

In virtue ethics, it is believed that who we are (and have been) predicts how we will act in the future – a presumption that is commonly manifested in society, whether in discussions about political candidates or in assessments of professional behavior. Take, for example, the kinds of character traits used to assess medical trainees: we look for reliability, diligence, thoroughness, sensitivity, altruism, compassion, and honesty. Such traits are virtues, and their assessment represents an evaluation of a person's character. By taking character seriously, we take virtue ethics seriously, and in so doing we express our belief that there is a reliable connection between who we are and what we do. The need to take character seriously in medicine is heightened by the awareness that what happens between patients and physicians is highly interpersonal, hidden from public view, and predicated on a physician's trustworthiness. Having the right kind of character increases the likelihood that a physician will act habitually in the interests of his patients, regardless of the circumstances and without concern for who may or may not be watching. Medical practice requires that we trust physicians not only to *know* what is right and good, but to have the *motivation* to do what is right and good as an expression of who they are as medical professionals. Such motivation is a matter of character.

B. Theory of Moral Value

The emphasis on persons and character in virtue ethics contrasts with the emphasis on principles or consequences in other approaches. Whereas principle-based theories place normative priority on actions that are claimed to be intrinsically right, and consequence-based theories hold that good outcomes are the criterion for determining which actions are right, virtue ethics takes the characteristic patterns of action of a virtuous moral agent as the primary source of normative value.[5] To appreciate the different ethical emphases that principles, consequences, and virtues bring to ethical deliberations, consider the challenge of disclosing medical errors. Imagine that a physician is caring for a patient hospitalized with pneumonia, and the physician inadvertently orders a drug at a dose that is two times greater than the appropriate amount. The next day there is evidence that this overdose has caused harm to the function of the patient's kidneys, but without causing any symptoms. The patient seems quite unaware that anything wrong has occurred. Because the mistake was

[5] Robert B. Louden, "On some vices of virtue ethics," *American Philosophical Quarterly* 21, no. 3 (1984): 228–29.

caught early, the physician expects the problem with kidney function to last only one or two days; but to be sure, she decides it will be necessary to add an extra day or two to the patient's hospitalization so the patient's condition can be monitored. Since there will likely be no lasting harm from the mistake and since the additional hospital days could be explained as giving the patient more time to heal, the physician wonders whether to tell the patient exactly what happened. If the physician were guided primarily by *principles* that included the obligation to tell the truth, she would be duty-bound to explain in a straightforward way what had happened, notwithstanding the negative repercussions that might result from disclosing the error. If the physician were guided primarily by *consequences,* she would try to identify the anticipated positive and negative effects of disclosing the error and then would disclose or not disclose them depending on her prediction of the overall outcome for everyone concerned, including herself. If the physician were guided primarily by *virtues,* the desire to be honest would motivate her action, and she would take steps to explain in a straightforward way what had happened. Following a principle of truth telling, calculating consequences, or desiring to be honest – these are the kinds of contrasts that can result from different ethical approaches.

The focus on persons in virtue ethics is illustrated nicely by Aristotle's belief that moral guidance is to be found by consulting the judgment of a good person, one whose practical wisdom is appropriately sensitive to the circumstances at hand and whose motivations are proper.[6] Unlike Plato (429–347 B.C.E.), who accepted that universal rules of behavior were available to guide human action,[7] Aristotle had little to say about following rules, even though he considered rules to be part of moral reasoning, especially for learners as compared with experts.[8] Like Aristotle, Thomas Aquinas (1225–74) was apparently of the view that hard and fast moral rules are difficult to come by, making it necessary to rely on prudence, not rules, to determine what to do in any given circumstance – though he also believed in some absolute moral rules, such as the prohibition of killing innocent persons.[9]

[6] Jonathan Lear, *Aristotle: the desire to understand* (Cambridge: Cambridge University Press, 1988), 158.

[7] Douglas C. Langston, *Conscience and other virtues: from Bonaventure to MacIntyre* (University Park: Pennsylvania State University Press, 2001), 17.

[8] Julia Annas, *The morality of happiness* (Oxford: Oxford University Press, 1993), 108.

[9] Davies, *The thought of Thomas Aquinas,* 237.

For Aristotle, the ultimate good or final end (in Greek, *telos*) for human beings was happiness, or flourishing (in Greek, *eudaimonia*).[10] This flourishing signifies the end toward which humans naturally aim, for it represents the best life possible in the midst of limitations imposed by the diverse opportunities, capacities, and circumstances that define different lives. *Eudaimonia* therefore guides human desire, and its achievement constitutes the fulfillment of desire. For Aristotle, ethics was therefore motivated by the desire to live a fulfilled life, and the virtuous life constituted that fulfillment, rather than serving merely as a means to it.[11] Though Aquinas understood the final end for humans in supernatural terms, his thought included a similar dynamic in which a conception of the good life for human beings precedes an understanding of the virtues that, if lived out, will lead to the achievement of that good life.[12] All moral action, for Aquinas, represents an attraction to an end perceived as good and a movement toward ultimate human fulfillment.[13]

A virtue-based framework along the lines of Aristotle or Aquinas raises questions about human nature and its fulfillment. These questions are controversial in a pluralistic society in which consensus about ultimate human ends is lacking. Yet some degree of social consensus about what constitutes human flourishing (and therefore virtue and vice) is a necessary provision for moral development. Children and other "moral learners" are expected to adopt the values of their community before they gain the ability to check those values against their individual understanding of virtue and vice based on experience and reflection.[14] But amid the moral pluralism of contemporary society, the existence of such shared communal values cannot be assumed.

In a morally pluralistic society, the lack of an agreed-upon final human end would appear to pose an insurmountable problem for virtue ethics, on the assumption that consensus about ultimate human purposes is necessary for agreement about the moral virtues that humans need in order to flourish. To the degree that our beliefs about ultimate human purposes shape our visions of the moral life and determine its virtues, there will necessarily be limits to the extent of common moral ground that can be encompassed by a virtue-based account of ethics.[15] We need to

10 Bostock, *Aristotle's ethics*, 11, 14.
11 Lear, *Aristotle: the desire to understand*, 155–57.
12 MacIntyre, *After virtue*, 184–85.
13 Davies, *The thought of Thomas Aquinas*, 227.
14 Annas, *The morality of happiness*, 113–14.
15 Meilaender, *The theory and practice of virtue*, 93.

remember these limits when we discuss virtue-based understandings of practical wisdom. But with this caution in mind, there are reasons to take virtue-based ethical approaches seriously for the contributions they offer to practical ethics. This is especially true in medicine because of the broad, albeit incomplete, consensus in the profession and society about the beliefs, values, virtues, and goals that should guide the work of health professionals. How extensive this consensus is, and how numerous its fracture lines from serious moral disagreements may be, are among the central concerns of this book.

C. Defining Moral Virtues

Although definitions vary as to exactly what a virtue is,[16] there is relatively broad agreement that virtues of moral significance are acquired traits or dispositions that make a person inclined to perform "certain kinds of actions in certain kinds of situations."[17] As an acquired rather than inherited quality, a virtue is learned by the practice of the very kinds of actions one would perform if one already had that virtue (e.g., one becomes generous by performing generous acts).[18] More broadly, virtues constitute the elements of moral character, and thereby help determine who we are as persons and create the moral lens through which we see the world.[19] As noted in Chapter 1, virtues also enable us to achieve the goods that are internal to a moral practice such as medicine and serve to define relationships between fellow participants in that practice.[20]

The ancient Greeks understood a virtue (in Greek, *arête*) to be an excellence, that is, the ability to do something excellently.[21] To have virtue in general was to have what was needed to live an excellent life.[22] For Aristotle, the virtues are "motivated dispositional states which aim at their own exercise: and the exercise of the virtues is constitutive of the good life for humans,"[23] by which human desires are organized in the pursuit of a truly happy life.[24] Aristotle's understanding of virtue also

[16] Edmund L. Pincoffs, "Two cheers for Meno: the definition of the virtues," in *Virtue and medicine*, ed. Earl E. Shelp (Dordrecht: Reidel, 1985), 111–31.
[17] Frankena, *Ethics*, 63.
[18] Lear, *Aristotle: the desire to understand*, 165–66.
[19] Meilaender, *The theory and practice of virtue*, 11.
[20] MacIntyre, *After virtue*, 191.
[21] Lear, *Aristotle: the desire to understand*, 153.
[22] Ibid., 164.
[23] Ibid., 186.
[24] Ibid., 164.

includes an affective (emotional) element, since to possess a virtue is to be disposed to have certain feelings in certain situations that, when combined with appropriate reasoning, lead to certain actions.[25] Accordingly, having a virtue entails a harmony between certain feelings and thoughts, with the result that a virtuous person enjoys doing what is virtuous. Julia Annas summarizes the ancient Greek understanding of the integration of the virtuous person's character and feelings in this way: "having a virtue is having one's character developed in such a way that one not only grasps what the right thing to do is but takes pleasure in doing it; one is repelled by the thought of wrong acting; and one is not seriously tempted by incentives not to do the right action."[26] Following Aristotle, Aquinas described virtues as habits that perfect human beings so that they act well[27] and as good dispositions that incline us "to act in ways that conduce to our flourishing, to our functioning to our best advantage, so that our needs as people are satisfied."[28]

D. Motivation and Intention

A key aspect of virtue is motivation. To possess a virtue is also to possess the motivation to act on it, so that the moral substance of the virtue is expressed through word or deed. Whether referred to as intention, will, or desire, this intrinsic motivational aspect of virtue distinguishes it from ethical approaches based on principles or consequences.[29] In the absence of moral motivation, there is less reason to believe that *knowing* what is good or right will lead to *doing* it. Virtue ethics bridges the gap between knowing and doing by insisting that having appropriate intentions or attitudes is a necessary (though not sufficient) requirement of the moral life.[30] The significance of motivation in virtue ethics is notable in the face of moral dilemmas, that is, in cases where moral values or principles appear to be in conflict. Successfully engaging a dilemma requires motivation to persevere through moral tensions, make discerning judgments amid uncertainty, and avoid treating moral values in ways that minimize their tensions and uncertainties. As William Frankena observed, morality "cannot be content

[25] Bostock, *Aristotle's ethics*, 38.
[26] Annas, *The morality of happiness*, 55.
[27] McInerny, "Ethics," 203.
[28] Davies, *The thought of Thomas Aquinas*, 239.
[29] Louden, "On some vices of virtue ethics," 229.
[30] Philippa Foot, "Virtues and vices," in *Virtue ethics*, ed. Stephen Darwall (Oxford: Blackwell, 2003), 107–108.

with the letter of its law, but must foster in us the dispositions that will sustain us in the hour of decision when we are choosing between conflicting principles of prima facie duty or trying to revise our working rules of right or wrong."[31]

Motivation flows not only outward in word and action, but also inward in moral self-understanding. In Aristotle's conception, the motivation of the virtuous person represents a fundamental desire and intention to live a certain sort of life in which moral reflection facilitates understanding that, when acted upon, fulfills a desire that is so elemental as to be part of a person's identity.[32] We should note that the emphasis on motivation in virtue ethics resonates with accounts of moral action that tie intention to accountability – that is, the belief that what a person *intended* to do in a given situation should count significantly in the moral assessment of what actually happened in that situation.[33] Virtue ethics can be seen as taking intentions seriously while also recognizing the moral significance of the rightness or wrongness of actions and the goodness or badness of their consequences.

E. How Many Virtues Are There?

Edmund Pincoffs has discussed the challenges of enumerating the virtues, and his creation of a taxonomy containing sixty-five of them illustrates the diversity of character traits that can be categorized as virtues.[34] By describing such a wide range of potentially appealing virtues, Pincoffs encourages us to avoid reductionist tendencies that limit the core content of the moral life to a single virtue or small number of virtues, such as Kant's conscientiousness, Mill's benevolence, the ancient Greeks' cardinal virtues (practical wisdom, courage, temperance, and justice), or the church fathers' combination of the cardinal virtues with three theological ones (faith, hope, and love). Nevertheless, interest in specifying which virtues are most central in the moral life has a long history, suggesting a need to understand and promote the moral character traits that are believed to be most important.

One of the benefits of discussing different specifications of which virtues are most important is that different selections allow us to detect

[31] Frankena, *Ethics*, 66.
[32] Lear, *Aristotle: the desire to understand*, 189.
[33] MacIntyre, *After virtue*, 209.
[34] Pincoffs, "Two cheers for Meno."

contrasts and tensions between different values. This is illustrated, for instance, by MacIntyre's comparison of Aristotelian and Christian values. He points out that the New Testament praises virtues (faith, hope, and love) of which Aristotle said nothing, ignores virtues (e.g., *phronesis*) that were crucial for Aristotle, and praises at least one virtue (humility) that Aristotle seemed to consider a vice (relative to magnanimity).[35] Comparisons also allow us to discern virtues that have stood time's testing – such as the four cardinal virtues, which can be seen as representing a moral consensus about the habits required for members of society to cooperate in the tasks of civil life. As Peter Geach observed, practical wisdom is needed for any large-scale planning; justice is needed to ensure cooperation and mutual trust; temperance, to avoid distraction by short-term satisfactions that interfere with long-term, large-scale goals; and courage, to persevere in the face of difficulty and danger.[36]

F. Unity of the Virtues

Another question involves the relationship of one virtue with another. Are the virtues mutually dependent on each other? Does a person have to possess all the virtues in order to possess any one of them? Put another way, does a person have to possess all the virtues to live a virtuous life? Although this may seem an overly theoretical question, it is a concrete concern in virtue ethics that can be prompted by the recognition, in our own lives and in the lives of others, that some virtues are more present than others. And it becomes an especially lively question when articulated in terms of so-called character flaws that detract from an otherwise admirable moral life. As an example in the context of medicine, if I am exemplary in the virtue of honesty but do rather poorly when it comes to the virtue of compassion, can I be considered a virtuous physician? Aristotle would have said no, for he believed that there is a unity to the virtues in the life of the virtuous person because one cannot have one virtue without having them all.[37] Similarly, Aquinas believed that the virtues "grow all together, proportionately like a man's fingers," even though a given virtue "may be more or less perfectly expressed."[38] But the claims of Aristotle and Aquinas can be challenged by the common observation that

[35] MacIntyre, *After virtue*, 182.

[36] Peter Geach, *The virtues* (Cambridge: Cambridge University Press, 1977), 16.

[37] Aristotle, *Nicomachean ethics*, trans. Martin Ostwald (Indianapolis: Bobbs-Merrill Educational Publishing, 1962), 172.

[38] Aquinas, *Summa theologica*, 244.

there are persons whose moral characteristics are admirable in some ways and faulty in others.

A further aspect of the question of the unity of the virtues involves the moral dilemmas that may arise from competing virtues. Are such conflicts between virtues real, or are they merely apparent and amenable to resolution through diligence and discernment? Geach suggests that all the virtues are mutually compatible[39] and that the experience of conflicting virtues – such as feeling compelled to lie in order to avoid some evil or harm – is due not to an in-built potential for tragic conflict among the virtues, but to a lack of wisdom regarding how different virtues are to be expressed in a given circumstance.[40] Rosalind Hursthouse is less certain about this, remaining open to the possibility that virtue ethics holds the same potential for genuine moral dilemmas (due to competing virtues) as principle-based ethics does (due to competing principles).[41] Gilbert Meilaender believes – and I think he is correct – that one's response to questions about the unity and potential for conflict among the virtues depends on how one envisions the moral life, that is, whether one sees the virtues as individual qualities that can exist in isolation or sees them as constituents of a harmonious moral life that is like "a seamless robe which must either be worn intact or not at all."[42] Seen as "a seamless robe," a life of virtue is not merely an episodic or concatenated expression of one moral quality after another, but a lifelong project of integration, in which virtues form and express a person's character and identity over time.

The relationship between different virtues is of particular significance for practical wisdom, because wisdom depends on other virtues, especially the other cardinal virtues. *Practical wisdom* shows us the good we need to pursue, but we also need *courage* to persevere in the pursuit of that good when facing risk or opposition; we need *temperance* (self-control) to stay our course when tempted by our own preferences or pleasures; and we need *justice* to treat each person impartially and as having equal worth. Because virtues are interdependent in the moral life, we can begin to appreciate how *integrity* – with its connotation of moral *integration* – is part of practical wisdom. By practical wisdom we may perceive a path forward, but we also need courage, temperance, and justice to proceed steadily down that path.

39 Geach, *The virtues*, 162.

40 Ibid., 121.

41 Rosalind Hursthouse, "Normative virtue ethics," in *Virtue ethics*, ed. Darwall, 193–98.

42 Meilaender, *The theory and practice of virtue*, 20.

However inviting and compelling virtue ethics may be, some of its features pose serious questions, particularly in the context of medical practice and training. The most significant question pertains to its need for a concept of human flourishing that provides a full picture of the kind of life the virtues are meant to achieve. Any efforts to reach consensus on what counts as human flourishing will be challenged by controversies about human nature and its purpose within a morally pluralistic profession and society. A second area of concern involves what we can call normative traction: Can the virtues provide a means of moral reasoning and communication capable of explaining and justifying ethical decision making? And third, virtue ethics poses important educational challenges that bear directly on medical training.

II. CHALLENGES FOR A VIRTUE-BASED UNDERSTANDING OF PRACTICAL WISDOM

A. Human Flourishing

Jonathan Lear describes how central the end (*telos*) of human life is to Aristotle's ethics and wherein this end is to be found.[43] Aristotle held that if there is an end to a person's activities, this must be the person's chief good; and a chief good is necessary to orient and subordinate all the various ends that are pursued in the course of a person's day or life. The chief good in human life is happiness, or flourishing (*eudaimonia*), in the same way that the chief good in medicine is health. For Aristotle, human happiness depends on what is uniquely human and on living a life that expresses that unique nature. The realization of this nature is therefore the chief good, or end, for human beings.

Some modern philosophers object that Aristotle's ethics depends on an outdated metaphysical biology and deny that humans have natures in which ethics can be grounded. One example is David Bostock, who describes Aristotle's biological teleology as an inductive argument based on the belief that human beings have a function and that a being's good is to be found in the realization of its function.[44] Aristotle's philosophy assumes that this function constitutes human nature, which fundamentally involves the ability to reason. Bostock does not accept Aristotle's biological teleology or his presumption that species and their natures

[43] Lear, *Aristotle: the desire to understand*, 160–68.

[44] Bostock, *Aristotle's ethics*, 225.

are fixed, and he argues against such presumptions in humans on the basis of cultural differences throughout the world. Bostock dismisses the notion of a universal human nature and invites his readers to consider what, if anything, can serve as a foundation for ethics, if human nature cannot.[45] Lear, however, believes that such objections are too strong and suggests that an Aristotelian understanding of human flourishing can help us understand human nature and the ethics appropriate to that nature. According to Lear;

> An ethical theory that is at least Aristotelian in inspiration need only believe that there are ways in which human beings can flourish which are recognizably ethical. One need only believe that human life is distinctive and potentially worthwhile; that there are certain ways of life that are fulfilling and rich and others that are degrading and deprived; that there are ways of living a cooperative, ethical life within society that are fulfilling and rich.[46]

Aquinas employs a variation of Aristotle's functional argument and concludes that what uniquely characterizes human beings is their ability to reason and to will, and the ultimate end for human beings – in their reasoning, willing, and acting – is their good.[47] For Aquinas, this good is found in God alone and, derivatively, in all that God has created.[48] Whereas Aristotle defines the end for human beings as flourishing, Aquinas describes it as blessedness (in Latin, *beatitudo*) – the complete happiness that comes from spiritual union with God through knowing, enjoying, and loving God.[49] Like Aristotle, Aquinas believes that human nature is the proper grounding for ethics, and he does so because he believes that human nature is created by God and, as such, is good. Brian Davies summarizes Aquinas as believing that "human goodness lies in acting in harmony with what people are by nature insofar as reason can discern this" and that our primary ethical imperative as human beings is to "recognize what we are and to act accordingly."[50]

For both Aristotle and Aquinas, ethics depends fundamentally on a view of human purpose that derives from an understanding of human nature. In our morally pluralistic society, diverse beliefs about human purpose and nature impede consensus about such dependence. This diversity also extends to interpretations of virtue-based approaches to ethics, resulting

45 Ibid., 27–29.
46 Lear, *Aristotle: the desire to understand*, 191.
47 McInerny, "Ethics," 200–202.
48 Davies, *The thought of Thomas Aquinas*, 229.
49 Ibid., 230.
50 Ibid., 231.

in different perspectives on the purpose of human life within an ethics of virtue. One suggestion, by Annas, is that happiness can be understood as a "thin" specification of human purpose that requires individual elaboration by each person based on his or her own beliefs:

> The ethics of virtue ... takes shape within the framework of a search for an adequate specification of my final end. In ancient ethics this is the entry point to serious ethical reflection; it is taken to be a deep fact about us that we do have such a final end and that when we start reflecting on our lives we do not rest until we have brought the whole of our lives into reflective focus. Further, it is taken for granted that this final end is happiness, though happiness is understood weakly and in an unspecific way.[51]

Another approach, illustrated by Geach, focuses not on ultimate ends, but on intermediate ones. He believes that intermediate ends can still allow us to think teleologically using Aristotelian principles about what human beings are for, without referring to obsolete notions of human biology.[52] In this way, we can achieve considerable agreement about the need for virtues such as practical wisdom, courage, temperance, and justice, without insisting on agreement about ultimate ends. Geach illustrates his point with reference to health care:

> Consider the fact that people of different religions or of no religion at all can agree to build and run a hospital, and agree broadly on what shall be done in the hospital. There will of course be marginal policy disagreements, e.g. about abortion operations and the limits of experimentation on human beings. But there can be agreement on fighting disease, because disease impedes men's efforts towards most goals.[53]

Geach's assessment rightly suggests that in contexts such as health care, placing virtues within a framework defined by broadly shared intermediate ends can accomplish a considerable amount of moral work. He is also right to point out that we disagree about some things only against a background of agreement about other things[54] and that the degree of our cooperation indicates the extent of our consensus about intermediate ends. In the setting of the hospital, compromises between diverse people are possible so long as their disagreements about the implications of ultimate ends are not too disruptive. (He notes, for example, that a Christian Scientist would not even support the existence of a hospital.) Yet even as

[51] Annas, *The morality of happiness.*
[52] Geach, *The virtues*, 12.
[53] Ibid., 13.
[54] Ibid., 14.

we rightly focus on shared intermediate ends, we should not lose sight of the ineliminable role that ultimate ends play in our moral assessments. This is especially important to remember, because virtues are tied to these ultimate ends and establish the moral conditions that make cooperation possible among persons with contrasting beliefs.[55]

B. Normative Justification

Critics of virtue ethics question whether virtues provide a basis to justify right action in practical decision making. In particular, they are concerned that virtue ethics lacks the kind of normative traction that principles and consequences are believed to have. As an illustration of such concerns, Robert Louden lists five reasons to object to virtue theory as an independent basis for normative ethics:

1. Virtue theory relies upon assessments of what a hypothetical virtuous person would do in a given set of circumstances and derives "oughts" (principles and rules) from these assessments; however, it is not always easy to determine what a virtuous person would do, and the derived "oughts" are often too vague to be helpful to persons who have not yet acquired the sensitivities and insights of a virtuous person.
2. Virtue theory is unable to explain how even the most virtuous people may make wrong choices.
3. Virtue theory is unable to justify absolute moral prohibitions for actions that are considered intolerable (not just bad), because of its normative reliance on characteristic patterns of behavior in virtuous persons.
4. Virtues are acquired as character develops, but moral sensitivities can be lost as well as gained and their susceptibility to flux implies that a more reliable moral standard is needed to gauge the quality of a person's moral life.
5. Emphasis on persons (rather than actions) runs the risk of excusing bad actions as temporary aberrations or "acts out of character."[56]

A key concern for Louden is that virtue theory cannot shake off doubts about our ability to determine which persons are virtuous and consequently fails to provide a meaningful account of virtues and vices

[55] Ibid., 20.
[56] Louden, "On some vices of virtue ethics."

themselves.[57] Bostock strikes a similarly critical note by arguing that Aristotle fails to provide a rational basis to justify a virtue as a virtue, and he concludes that the determination of an Aristotelian virtue is more a matter of habituation than of reason.[58]

In the face of such criticisms, defenders of virtue ethics offer various explanations in an attempt to justify the conclusion that virtues can provide normative grounding for ethical decision making. Pincoffs, for example, suggests that virtues represent our habits of responding to the persons around us, such that virtues and vices are "dispositional properties that provide grounds for preference or avoidance of persons."[59] Instead of resting the weight of justification for virtues on a shared understanding of human flourishing, Pincoffs identifies the choices of the moral agent as the locus of moral justification: preferences establish virtues, and avoidances establish vices. But this descriptive strategy leaves us wondering what sorts of persons ought to be preferred or avoided and why. His approach seems unlikely to do more than reflect prevailing social conventions.

In responding to the problem of normative traction, Julia Annas acknowledges the dependence of virtue ethics on social convention by conceding the need for some appeal to consensus to determine what constitutes a given virtue. She believes that judgments about right action are derived neither from the virtuous agent nor from some independent objective standpoint. Instead there is a process of "reflective equilibrium" between "the virtuous person's viewpoint and society's consensus" that allows the novice in virtue to be nurtured by the shared views of others.[60] Annas also explains that the ancients did not attempt to be hierarchical or complete in their portrayals of the moral life,[61] and they did not contemplate the possibility of radical moral error in their understanding about which dispositions were virtuous or vicious, since they believed that the virtues are natural to us, based on general truths about human nature.[62]

References to ancient Greece in discussions about virtue ethics raise questions about the extent to which the moral framework of one culture can be transposed to another. Louden argues that it is problematic

57 Ibid., 232–33.

58 Bostock, *Aristotle's ethics*, 100.

59 Pincoffs, "Two cheers for Meno," 114.

60 Annas, *The morality of happiness*, 113–14.

61 Ibid., 111.

62 Ibid., 115.

to appropriate a framework derived from the moral homogeneity of Aristotle's ancient Greek culture and apply it to the moral heterogeneity of contemporary society. Seeking guidance from virtuous persons to determine the definition and application of the virtues may have made sense in Aristotle's Greece, but not amid the pluralism of modern societies, he maintains. Louden believes that it is simply untenable to base normative conclusions about virtues on guidance from persons deemed virtuous given how widely members of modern societies disagree about moral values. Louden fears that this is what contemporary virtue ethicists have mistakenly attempted to do.[63]

Another defender of virtue ethics, Rosalind Hursthouse, offers a lengthy defense of its capacity for normative traction. She contends that virtue ethics stands as a normative rival to principle-based or consequence-based approaches by its ability to provide guiding rules: there is, she contends, one positive rule for each virtue and one prohibition for each vice. Furthermore, she argues that virtue ethics not only makes reference to persons and their characters, but can also specify right action, as follows: "An action is right [if and only if] it is what a virtuous agent would characteristically (i.e. acting in character) do in the circumstances."[64] Hursthouse also argues that in responding to the challenge of normative traction, approaches based on principles, consequences, or virtues are all under the same burden to justify a source of normative guidance that precedes the particular method each approach employs. Principle-based accounts have to specify what counts as a correct principle, consequence-based accounts have to specify what counts as the best consequence, and virtue-based accounts have to specify who counts as a virtuous moral agent. On the basis of the availability of rules that correlate with each virtue, she also objects to the claim that virtue ethics is incompatible with moral absolutes, citing examples of virtue ethicists (including Aquinas) who have held certain rules, such as "Do not lie," to be absolute prohibitions.[65]

Hursthouse's argument that virtue ethics is on a par with principle-based and consequence-based approaches in their shared need for normative justification is well taken. Yet her need to translate virtues into rules in order to establish a means of determining right action reveals the pride of place that principles seem to hold in contemporary ethics. This priority is affirmed by Frankena, who maintains that we ultimately

[63] Louden, "On some vices of virtue ethics," 233.
[64] Hursthouse, "Normative virtue ethics," 187.
[65] Rosalind Hursthouse, *On virtue ethics* (Oxford: Oxford University Press, 1999), 85.

judge an action right or wrong by reference to a principle or set of principles,[66] a point reinforced by the observation that even when actions are assessed on consequentialist grounds, their merits are based on a principle (e.g., the principle of utility). Yet Frankena also reminds us that virtue ethics brings *intention* to morality, allowing us to understand how an agent's intention or motive can affect the goodness or badness of an action regardless of its outcome – that is, one can inadvertently do the right thing for evil reasons.[67]

The challenge of establishing normative grounding in virtue ethics leads some of its proponents to embrace the need for deeper sources of justification and integration with other ethical approaches. For instance, Pellegrino and Thomasma maintain that virtue ethics ought to be anchored in a theory of morality and human nature, sustained by a community of practice, and linked conceptually with duties, rules, and consequences.[68] By acknowledging the need to complement virtues with duties and rules, Pellegrino and Thomasma recognize the importance of placing virtue ethics in a larger theoretical context, such as one finds in natural law and its assumption that there are moral starting points, or principles, accessible to all persons. In Aquinas's natural law philosophy, for example, such principles communicate rock-bottom goods and unassailable truths to which all people have access even if they do not have a theory of natural law. For Aquinas, examples of such principles would include exceptionless prohibitions against lying, theft, and adultery – which, he believed, all people are capable of recognizing.[69] The need for principles of right action to establish normative boundaries for virtuous behavior implies that virtues and principles should be viewed neither in isolation nor in competition, but in a complementary relationship of integration.

C. Education

A third major challenge for virtue ethics involves moral education. As acquired traits, virtues are learned, and they come much more through experience and practice in real situations than through lectures or discussions in seminar rooms. How medical educators are supposed to "educate" trainees in virtue is therefore a pressing question, and the pedagogical

66 Frankena, *Ethics*, 70.

67 Ibid.

68 Edmund D. Pellegrino and David C. Thomasma, *The virtues in medical practice* (New York: Oxford University Press, 1993), 190.

69 McInerny, "Ethics," 212–13.

challenges that exist for all the moral virtues are perhaps even more daunting in the case of practical wisdom. As Aristotle observed, young people may become good mathematicians, but they do not attain practical wisdom, for "practical wisdom is concerned with particulars as well <as with universals>, and knowledge of particulars comes from experience."[70] Aquinas similarly observed that the acquisition of prudence "needs time and experience, so the young have it neither in act nor in disposition."[71] Annas describes the acquisition of virtue as a process of habituation through reflective practice and affective development by which a person's attitudes evolve and her feelings become more in tune with her deliberative judgments.[72] A learner of practical wisdom first depends on rules and deliberation and then gains expertise, which is accompanied by the skill of quickly discerning the morally relevant features of any situation.[73]

Desire, argues Lear, is a crucial element for training in virtue because the task of ethical education "is not to get us to perform noble acts even though our desires pull us toward bad things, but rather to reorganize our desires so that we get pleasure from doing noble acts and pain from doing bad ones."[74] The need for "reorganized desires" is perhaps clearest for those who are young and need to be cajoled into virtue through appropriate encouragements and discouragements rather than through rational persuasion.[75] For adults, education in virtue is – somewhat paradoxically – for people who already have the desire to be virtuous and thereby are, to that extent, already leading a virtuous life. Notably, Aristotle's purpose in the *Nicomachean Ethics* was not to persuade its readers to become virtuous or to show them how, but to assist them in their moral self-understanding so that they could develop a more coherent ethical outlook.[76] Aristotle's assessment that virtue is a prerequisite for advancing in virtue sounds a cautionary note for those who might be too optimistic about the prospects for training adult learners in virtue.

Another way of describing how growth in virtue depends on desire is to say that moral training requires a learner to delight in what is good. In Greek, medieval, and Renaissance cultures, this kind of learning was typically accomplished by storytelling, which served as the chief means

70 Aristotle, *Nicomachean ethics*, 160.
71 Aquinas, *Summa theologica*, 378.
72 Annas, *The morality of happiness*, 58.
73 Ibid., 91.
74 Lear, *Aristotle: the desire to understand*, 168.
75 Ibid., 189–90.
76 Ibid., 157–59.

of moral education through the communication of moral images and exemplars that would awaken in the listener a love for what is good and, thereby, help shape the character of the listener.[77] Within a framework of virtue, the shaping of a person's character is a matter not of transferring knowledge, but of seeking a vision of the good within a supportive community that encourages its members to delight in what is good.[78]

The need for a moral community that cultivates virtue warrants particular attention in the context of medical training. Authors such as Pellegrino and Thomasma believe that virtue can be taught by various means, such as personal practice, the example of others, and the study of ethics. However, their expectations are modest.[79] The stronger claim they and others make is that the training environment is inevitably influential, and highly so, whether for the enhancement of virtue or for its corrosion. Medical educators cannot avoid contributing to this environment, for better or worse.[80] This is a critical concern in medical training that has in recent years been discussed as a problem of the so-called hidden curriculum. This "under-the-radar" reality comprises aspects of the interpersonal and institutional learning environment that embody negative values which learners deem practically useful and therefore important; these negative values are therefore internalized, even though they contradict the positive values of the formal curriculum.[81]

Professional communities inevitably communicate moral values through the words and behaviors of their members. On the assumption that these values have the potential to influence the moral development of trainees, those responsible for training in ethics and professionalism need always to consider how to make the training environment as virtue-enhancing as possible. This is the rationale that leads Pellegrino and Thomasma to conclude that medical school faculty members have a de facto obligation to take at least some responsibility for the character formation of their trainees.[82]

A virtue-based understanding of training recognizes that learners grow in virtue through imitation, which explains why a supportive community of practice is vital to character formation. Imitation is essential

77 Meilaender, *The theory and practice of virtue*, 54–55.

78 Ibid., 68–72.

79 Pellegrino and Thomasma, *The virtues in medical practice*, 176.

80 Ibid., 179.

81 F. W. Hafferty and R. Franks, "The hidden curriculum, ethics teaching, and the structure of medical education," *Academic Medicine* 69 (1994): 861–71.

82 Pellegrino and Thomasma, *The virtues in medical practice*, 180.

in virtue theory because it is understood that a person becomes virtuous by practicing virtuous behaviors. Imitating a virtue is viewed as practicing a skill in order to master it or playing a role in order to enter into it. Advocates of virtue ethics realize that it may seem disingenuous, even hypocritical, to counsel learners to become virtuous (gain the proper feelings associated with virtue) by practicing virtue (while not yet having those proper feelings). But the suggestion of hypocrisy is based on the mistaken assumption that imitation implies insincerity. It need not do so. A person can imitate a virtue for many reasons, not all of which are virtuous. But if someone imitates a virtue in order to become more virtuous, there is a sincerity to the imitation that derives from an underlying intention. As Meilaender describes it, imitating virtue is like putting on a mask, "not with any intention to dissemble, but in the hope that we may gradually begin to look more like the mask, in the hope that our feelings may gradually conform to our behavior."[83] Sincere imitation of virtue can reflect the hope that our deeper desires can be expressed in the willingness to practice behaviors that we wish were part of our character but are not yet so. Imitation of virtue is a stage en route to moral maturity. In this sense, the virtues are like other skills that are observed and copied before they are internalized and possessed.

A final educational question for virtue ethics concerns the need for consensus within an educational environment concerning what constitutes virtue (and what constitutes vice). As previously noted, Annas recognizes the need for some appeal to consensus to establish the domain of virtue in society, a domain from which individuals start in their moral development and with which they constructively engage as they advance in self-reflection and mature in virtue. With respect to medical training, Pellegrino and Thomasma are more definite, maintaining that moral consensus, within medical schools and the medical profession, is essential to sustain the practices of virtuous physicians.[84] We should note that moral consensus can be manifested in words, practices, or policies. Sometimes the institutional, regulatory, and economic structures in which physicians practice and trainees learn can be as influential as formal pronouncements regarding professional ethical standards. For example, structural realities in hospital services and clinic schedules may teach trainees that efficiency and economic productivity are valued more than respect for patients' questions, sensitivity to their anxieties, or compassion for their suffering.

[83] Meilaender, *The theory and practice of virtue*, 78.
[84] Pellegrino and Thomasma, *The virtues in medical practice*, 180.

And pressures of time, requirements for billing, and demands for information to satisfy quality metrics may lead to superficial documentation practices that teach trainees that the electronic medical record is more a means to economic and regulatory ends than a source of meaningful information that documents and facilitates patient care.

III. COMPARING ETHICAL APPROACHES BASED ON VIRTUES, PRINCIPLES, AND CONSEQUENCES

Earlier in this chapter virtue ethics was briefly contrasted with other ethical approaches that focus on principles or consequences, and questions about the comparative ability of virtue ethics to gain moral traction have been considered. Because of the interrelationships between different ethical approaches, it is useful to consider in more detail how a virtue-based framework compares with frameworks based on principles or consequences. The importance of this comparison arises both from the multifaceted nature of moral experience and from a practical and educational need to understand why virtue ethics is a vital complement to these other frameworks.

In comparing virtue-based and principle-based frameworks, it is notable that proponents of each approach are ready to recognize that whatever their differences may be, there is an intimate relationship between the two frameworks. As previously mentioned, Hursthouse maintains that virtue ethics is composed of moral dispositions (virtues and vices) that can be translated into rules (positive and negative) that specify right action. Seen this way, virtues can be understood as having the capacity to function like principles.[85] Frankena believes that it is important to appreciate the difference between a principle and a virtue, but he nevertheless recognizes that the relationship between principles and virtues is so close that each could properly be recast as the other.[86] Such accounts suggest it is unnecessary to treat principle-based and virtue-based frameworks as rivals, since they can reasonably be considered complementary aspects of the same morality. As summarized by Frankena, "for every principle there will be a morally good trait, often going by the same name, consisting of a disposition or tendency to act according to it; and for every morally good

[85] Hursthouse, "Normative virtue ethics," 187–93.

[86] Frankena, *Ethics*, 63–64. Frankena suggests that his theory of obligation, founded on the principles of beneficence and justice, could be recast in virtue terms employing the dispositions of benevolence and justice (the latter being the disposition to treat people equally).

trait there will be a principle defining the kind of action in which it is to express itself."[87] And the complementarity between virtues and principles does not mean they lack distinctive features. In a virtue-based framework, the virtues play a dual role of instruction and motivation; in a principle-based framework, instruction is provided by the normative power of principles and motivation comes from the virtues. The most important role of the virtues in an ethics of principles is to provide the motivation to willingly follow the guidance that principles provide.[88] Frankena offers a pithy summary of the complementarity of principles and virtues when he suggests that principles without virtues are powerless, and virtues without principles are blind.[89]

An appreciation for the complementary values of virtues and principles is also provided by Tom Beauchamp and James Childress.[90] They perceive a vital correspondence between the four principles of biomedical ethics (beneficence, nonmaleficence, respect for autonomy, and justice) and their corollary virtues (benevolence, nonmalevolence, respectfulness, and justice). Indeed, they suggest that there is an extensive range of correlated principles (or rules) and virtues, even though a one-to-one correspondence does not exist for all principles and virtues (sometimes because a given virtue, such as courage or integrity, is important for morality as a whole and not just for one principle or rule). Beauchamp goes so far as to suggest that principles of duty and virtue standards can "in principle be conceived as in a relation of perfect correspondence," such that every principle has a corresponding character trait (the disposition to act as the principle specifies).[91] Beauchamp also argues that the correspondence between virtues and principles can be wedded to the correlativity theory of rights and duties (the right of one person entails a duty in another, and vice versa), the implication being that the correlation between virtues and principles also extends to rights. In this way, Beauchamp wants to draw our attention to a fundamental relationship between three basic aspects of morality: virtue standards, principles of duty, and rights.[92] Like Frankena, Beauchamp grants priority to principles,

[87] Ibid., 65.
[88] Ibid., 67.
[89] Ibid., 65.
[90] Tom L. Beauchamp and James F. Childress, *Principles of biomedical ethics*, 6th ed. (New York: Oxford University Press, 2009), 45–46.
[91] Tom L. Beauchamp, "What's so special about the virtues?" in *Virtue and medicine*, ed. Shelp, 311.
[92] Ibid., 316.

on the grounds that virtues cannot serve as primary action guides or as primary sources of moral appraisal. Nevertheless, he appreciates the irreplaceable value of virtues and commends complementarity: "A morality of principles of duty should enthusiastically recommend settled dispositions to act in accordance with that which is morally required, and a proponent of virtue ethics should encourage the development of principles that express how one ought to act."[93]

In contrast to the friendly relationship between virtue-based and principle-based ethical approaches, the relationship between virtue-based and consequence-based approaches is more likely to be viewed as a rivalry. As Hursthouse explains in the course of discussing absolute moral prohibitions, "virtue ethicists and deontologists tend to stand shoulder to shoulder against utilitarians, denying that, for example, this lie can be told, this promise broken, this human being killed because the consequences of so doing will be generally happiness-maximizing."[94] Annas addresses this contrast by referring to Sidgwick's belief that commonsense morality is "explicitly deontological but implicitly consequentialist," meaning that we tend to acknowledge the force of moral principles, but we can be convinced by argument to see that underlying these principles is an intention to achieve good consequences.[95] As a result, principles can be seen as providing moral stability, while concern for predicted outcomes of action can be seen as providing flexibility and a willingness to modify the way principles are applied.

It seems unobjectionable to say that consequentialist reasoning is a common aspect of practical morality, particularly in the practice of medicine, where anticipated outcomes are so important for decision making. Predicted outcomes based on calculated benefits (of life and health) or risks (of suffering, disability, or death) are essential to moral analysis and therefore stand unavoidably alongside principles and virtues. But taking the anticipated balance of consequences seriously in a given patient's case is not the same as adopting consequentialism generally as a guiding conceptual framework in which a single principle (e.g., utility) defines a single good as the basic determinant of right action.

From the perspective of virtue ethics, two problems of consequentialist frameworks warrant particular attention. The first involves the inherent difficulty of predicting the future. This arises both from the unforeseeable

[93] Ibid., 310.

[94] Hursthouse, "Normative virtue ethics," 191–92.

[95] Annas, *The morality of happiness*, 454.

character of human affairs and medical outcomes and from the difficulty of deciding how far into the future one is obliged to extend one's predictions. As Geach acknowledges, the consequentialist might suggest that "one can ignore the consequences of an action after a certain time because they die out like ripples on a pond."[96] But Geach is not persuaded that consequentialism itself warrants such a conclusion. Instead, he looks to the virtue of practical wisdom, which equips a person to apply a "cut-off procedure" that places a reasonable limit on how far into the future the possible effects of an action must be considered and that also goes no farther into the future once an action is sufficiently described to identify it as intolerable (e.g., because it is an instance of killing the innocent, violating justice, etc.).

The second problem involves the nature of virtue and the goods that are internal to a practice, which is addressed by MacIntyre in two parts.[97] First, it can be argued that virtue must be practiced without inordinate regard for consequences, since to practice a virtue only on some occasions, on the basis of contingent circumstances, is to not possess that virtue at all. In this sense, virtue is genuinely independent of predicted consequences. Second, consequentialism is unable to support the distinction between goods internal to a practice and goods external to it. Because internal and external goods are incommensurable (i.e., they are not comparable on a single scale of measurement), it is not morally legitimate to homogenize them within the kinds of unidimensional moral calculations upon which consequentialist analyses depend. Moreover, we can extend this concern beyond MacIntyre's contrast between internal and external goods by pointing out that medicine, *within its internal goods*, also faces a challenge of incommensurability. Consider, for example, the context of end-of-life care, in which physicians and patients may sometimes struggle to balance the good of prolonging life against the good of providing comfort. Or consider how physicians, patients, and society can face the challenge of balancing the allocation of expensive resources to support one critically ill person against relatively inexpensive treatments to improve the health of many non-critically ill persons in the same community. There are some goods that, because of their contrasts, cannot legitimately be treated as if they were somehow amenable to comparison on a single scale of valuation. When comparing apples and oranges, people should not pretend that differences between fruits do not exist.

[96] Geach, *The virtues*, 100.

[97] MacIntyre, *After virtue*, 198–99.

These criticisms highlight some of the problems of consequentialism as a theoretical framework. Nevertheless, consequentialist considerations draw our attention to the moral significance of outcomes in ethical decision making, and they may suggest a tendency in virtue ethics to undervalue the importance of outcomes in ethical reasoning. Louden makes this point when arguing that both virtue-based and principle-based frameworks have weak notions of what he calls "product-ends" (the outcomes of actions) as opposed to the "activity-ends" (dutiful or virtuous activities) that produce them. Yet virtue ethics may not be as susceptible to this charge as Louden suggests, for virtue ethics involves an overarching teleological framework in which ends are crucial for orienting and guiding the process of moral reasoning. This is seen clearly in the virtue of practical wisdom, as will be discussed in the next chapter. In the context of medicine, we can express the teleological orientation of virtue ethics concretely by emphasizing the importance of goals of care. In this way, virtue ethics can be understood as requiring a goal-based means of assessing moral actions; and to the extent that actions aim at goals, virtue ethicists will be keenly interested in determining whether the consequences of action are likely to achieve those goals. Thus virtue ethics should not be viewed as neglecting outcomes, but rather as assessing both outcomes and the means used to achieve them by situating both outcomes and means within a multidimensional framework of values and goals. We can agree with MacIntyre and other virtue ethicists that the power and relevance of virtues is morally independent of consequences, and we can do so without risking the suggestion that virtue ethics does not take consequences seriously.

The preceding discussion of continuities and contrasts among virtues, principles, and consequences leads to a conclusion that is neither new nor surprising. An approach to ethical reasoning, if it is to reflect the traditions and practices of morality as we have come to understand them, has to be multifaceted. Among the three moral frameworks that have been discussed, the clearest line of demarcation separates consequentialist approaches from those based on virtues or principles. But if we can view consequentialist considerations modestly as a means of emphasizing the seriousness of outcomes in the moral life, the line of separation is perhaps more of conceptual interest than practical concern. Consistent with such a view, we can appreciate the need for inclusive approaches to contrasting frameworks. Louden, for instance, signals the interrelatedness of virtue-based, deontological, and consequentialist moral frameworks and marks the need for coordination between their complementary ethical approaches, on the belief that none of them alone is sufficient to explain morality as we understand it.[98] Pellegrino recognizes the need for a synthetic approach to an overarching framework of morality, emphasizing the importance of linking theories based on rights, duties, and virtues within a single theory of the good.[99] Beauchamp and Childress maintain that even though actions must be calibrated toward desired results and made to conform to relevant principles, "the goals and structure of medicine, health care, and research call for a deep appreciation of virtues"[100] – and they go so far as to say that there is no reason to consider principles superior to virtues or vice versa.[101] Beauchamp also speaks to the need for an "integrated theory of morality according to which virtue standards, principles of duty, and valid claims of right express different emphases in the moral life and are complementary categories,"[102] adding that the details of a given context will determine what is needed – whether it be blunt moral imperatives (rights), firmly formulated duties (principles), or persons of good character (virtues).[103]

The summary message promoted by such writers is that ethics requires a coordination and integration of its complementary approaches, and any tendencies toward conceptual rivalry should yield to cooperation. It is in this spirit of cooperation that virtue ethics in general, and the virtue of practical wisdom in particular, are discussed in this book.

IV. SUMMARY

Virtue ethics provides a framework in which the virtue of practical wisdom can be defined, related to other virtues, and contrasted with other approaches to ethics, such as those that rely primarily on principles or consequences. Principle-based (deontological) approaches emphasize duties of obligation and the rightness or wrongness of actions, such as killing or lying. Consequence-based (consequentialist or utilitarian) approaches emphasize the overall outcomes of actions and the goodness or badness of those outcomes, such as the consequences of killing or lying. By contrast, virtue-based approaches emphasize persons and the defining

98 Louden, "On some vices of virtue ethics."

99 Edmund D. Pellegrino, "The virtuous physician, and the ethics of medicine," in *Virtue and Medicine*, ed. Shelp, 248–50.

100 Beauchamp and Childress, *Principles of biomedical ethics*, 30–33.

101 Ibid., 57.

102 Beauchamp, "What's so special about the virtues?" 318.

103 Ibid., 324–25.

importance of the kind of persons we are and want to be, such as nonviolent or honest. Virtue ethics thereby directs our attention to being, without denying the importance of thinking and doing, and it assumes that who we are predicts how we will act, based on our moral character and the moral motivation that accompanies it.

Virtue ethics traditionally involves an understanding of a final end (*telos*) for human beings that is described as happiness or flourishing. What constitutes human flourishing is open to debate in a morally pluralistic society. But despite divergent assessments about ultimate human ends, virtue ethics holds particular potential for medicine, in which intermediate ends, like health and healing, enjoy broad consensus and provide a considerable amount of common moral ground.

Virtues are acquired traits of character that integrate thinking, feeling, motivation, and intention, and though virtues are many and variously categorized, historically significant listings include the cardinal virtues (practical wisdom, courage, temperance, and justice) and the theological virtues (faith, hope, and love). There is an interdependence between different virtues that is illustrated by the way practical wisdom both depends on and integrates other virtues – revealing a basic conceptual link between the virtue of practical wisdom and the idea of moral integrity (when it is taken to entail moral integration).

Education in virtue ethics is achieved not merely by instruction, but through experience, practice, and imitation, which allow moral attitudes, feelings, and judgments to grow together within a supportive community of fellow practitioners. Growth in virtue is predicated on the desire to be virtuous, which includes learning to delight in what is good, often through the sharing of stories whose narratives describe moral images and exemplars. The need for a moral community that can cultivate virtue is directly applicable to the context of medical training, especially in light of problems associated with the so-called hidden curriculum – the "under-the-radar" learning of negative values that contradict the positive values promoted by the formal curriculum. In order to help form the virtues of individual practitioners and trainees, medical communities require a substantial degree of moral consensus, which should be manifested not only in official words celebrating professional ideals, but also by practices, policies, and institutional structures that support those ideals.

There is a friendly complementarity between virtue-based and principle-based ethical approaches. Whereas principles provide the means to articulate normative direction for moral action, virtues identify character traits that motivate people to follow the direction that principles provide.

To highlight this contrast, it can be said that principles without virtues are powerless, and virtues without principles are blind. We can see the correlation between principles and virtues reflected in our language when we distinguish between, for example, the principle of *beneficence* and virtue of *benevolence*.

The relationship between virtue-based and consequence-based approaches to ethics is less friendly, since virtue ethics denies what formal consequentialist forms of ethical reasoning affirm, that different goods in the moral life – such as freedom, life, pleasure, and justice – can be treated as if commensurable on a single scale of measurement. Nevertheless, consequentialist considerations are justifiably ingrained in practical morality, especially in medicine, where ethical assessments necessarily incorporate the likely outcomes of different courses of action. Because of its ends-orientation (teleology), virtue ethics takes outcomes of actions seriously, as seen in the virtue of practical wisdom. In the context of medicine, this teleological orientation is particularly manifested through goals of care. Virtue ethics has the capacity to assess the value of outcomes, as well as the means used to achieve them, by situating both within a multidimensional framework of values and goals.

The complementarities and differences among virtue-based, principle-based, and consequence-based ethics encourage a multifaceted approach to ethical reasoning in which these three categories of moral values are integrated and prioritized. Tendencies toward conceptual rivalry among different ethical approaches should yield, whenever possible, to cooperation, and it is in such a spirit of cooperation that virtue ethics and practical wisdom are discussed in this book.

3

Practical Wisdom in Medicine

The task of a physician is to promote healing and preserve health by understanding and treating medical problems. Whether these problems are subjectively presented by the patient or objectively identified by the physician, they are the reason for the encounter between the patient and physician, and they are often challenging because of the complexity and variability with which illness is experienced, disease is expressed, and risks and benefits to health are assessed. In each patient, the physician encounters multiple dimensions of human existence (biological, psychological, social, spiritual), and decisions are often made amid unavoidable uncertainty due to incomplete diagnostic or prognostic information or because the preferences of patients or their surrogates are unclear. The demands of decision making that arise from these realities reflect the extent of a physician's need for practical wisdom.

Two central claims are put forth in this chapter: that practical wisdom in clinical medicine is fundamentally about the ability to know what ends or goals are worth pursuing and what means are most likely to achieve them, and that clinicians need practical wisdom in order to fulfill their obligation to care well for their patients as persons. To support these claims I draw from an understanding of practical wisdom based on frameworks of virtue ethics that trace back to Aristotle and Thomas Aquinas. In doing so I try to show how the virtue of practical wisdom resonates deeply with contemporary perceptions of the importance of goals of care in clinical decision making, and I suggest that an appreciation of this importance signifies a perceived need for practical wisdom in medicine. I also explore the close connection between practical wisdom in medicine and clinical judgment: both involve perceiving the reality of a patient's situation and responding to that reality in a health-promoting fashion. But while clinical judgment tends to be discussed in terms that focus on the biomedical tasks of diagnosis and treatment, practical wisdom adds an explicitly *ethical* dimension because wisdom requires that we appreciate what is good for a patient as a person, not merely as a biological being.

I. TRADITIONAL CONCEPTIONS OF PRACTICAL WISDOM: *PHRONESIS* AND *PRUDENTIA*

Within traditional frameworks of virtue developed by Aristotle and Aquinas, practical wisdom is the most important of the four cardinal virtues, since the other virtues depend on practical wisdom for their application. Whether referred to as *phronesis* in Greek (Aristotle) or *prudentia* in Latin (Aquinas), practical wisdom represents the ability to respond realistically and appropriately to a decision-making challenge, an ability that requires clear perception and integrated reasoning in response to a given set of circumstances. It is this rational engagement with a concrete reality external to the moral agent that explains the importance of practical wisdom for the other virtues, since a proper understanding of when and how those other virtues are to be expressed depends not merely on the moral agent's good intentions, but also on the objective features of a situation and the moral values that pertain to it. Practical wisdom supplies a discerning and deliberating rationality that perceives, considers, assesses, weighs, and so determines what course of action is warranted with respect to the circumstances at hand. We cannot detach the virtue of courage, for instance, from practical wisdom without depriving the moral agent of her appreciation of what courage might require in a given situation. That is why in a dangerous setting like a burning building, practical wisdom is required of firefighters and others so that they can decide whether an attempt to save a life would be an act of courage or foolishness.

The rational character of practical wisdom caused Aristotle and Aquinas to classify practical wisdom as an *intellectual virtue*,[1] as distinguished from *moral virtues* such as courage, temperance, and justice. Aristotle classified as intellectual those virtues of the soul that entailed reason, whereas the moral virtues were those that entailed feelings and required "listening to" reason.[2] This intellectual–moral distinction notwithstanding, in ancient and medieval thought there are very close connections between practical wisdom and the moral virtues, as the composition of cardinal virtues

[1] Foot, "Virtues and vices," 106.

[2] Bostock, *Aristotle's ethics*, 35.

demonstrates. Edmund Pellegrino and David Thomasma consider practical wisdom the link between the intellectual and moral virtues,[3] and Jonathan Lear captures the relationship neatly by saying that moral virtue "as it were, flows through the mind," since virtuous decisions are not automatically produced but require reasoning and conscious sensitivity to the details of a situation.[4] In passing it should be noted that, in Aristotle's philosophy, practical wisdom is distinguished from another intellectual virtue, *philosophical wisdom* (in Greek, *sophia*). Whereas practical wisdom pertains to practical thinking, political living, and the moral virtues, philosophical wisdom pertains to contemplation of the essence of things and basic truths about the structure of reality.[5]

For Aristotle, practical wisdom is the ability to perceive and act according to a proper understanding of the ends relevant to a situation by employing the proper means to achieve those ends.[6] It is a practical ability that identifies the right means to accomplish the right ends that virtue determines.[7] Julia Annas finds it difficult to translate Aristotle's *phronesis* into English and concludes that *practical intelligence* is the term probably most suitable for communicating the inventiveness and problem-solving character of "the disposition to make right moral judgments."[8] Lear underscores the significance of ends and means in Aristotle's practical wisdom, describing it as "a developed ability to judge the good and bad ends for man and to choose the actions appropriate for securing those ends in the particular circumstances of life."[9] Philippa Foot also emphasizes the ends–means relationship that characterizes practical wisdom when explaining that "the wise man knows the means to certain good ends; and secondly he knows how much particular ends are worth."[10] To this she adds the qualification that practical wisdom – in contrast to mere cleverness – applies only to *good* ends. Practical wisdom therefore involves normative evaluations of different possible ends, as well as decisions about which ends are most worthy of pursuit in a given context.[11] On this point, Aristotle observes that while the clever person has "the

[3] Pellegrino and Thomasma, *The virtues in medical practice*, 84.
[4] Lear, *Aristotle: the desire to understand*, 171–72.
[5] Ibid., 172–73.
[6] Aristotle, *Nicomachean ethics*, 152–58.
[7] Ibid., 169.
[8] Annas, *The morality of happiness*, 73.
[9] Lear, *Aristotle: the desire to understand*, 173.
[10] Foot, "Virtues and vices," 109.
[11] Ibid., 109–10.

power to perform those steps which are conducive to a goal," only the good person has the ability to judge those ends that are good, which is to say that only the person of virtue has practical wisdom.[12]

Though Aquinas was inspired by a Christian belief system and separated from Aristotle by more than 1,500 years, his understanding of practical wisdom and the other cardinal virtues was highly influenced by an Aristotelian framework.[13] Aquinas referred to practical wisdom as prudence and understood it to be the virtue that allows one to reason rightly about how to act by identifying the right means to accomplish the goals of moral virtue.[14] Prudence, according to Aquinas, "directs means to ends" through the deliberation of the mind and the choices made by the will.[15] The operation of prudence presupposes "the goals of moral virtue as general starting-points" and determines how they are to be applied in particular circumstances.[16] Aquinas argues that prudence and the other cardinal virtues are therefore mutually dependent.

> For we can't possess moral virtue without being prudent: since moral virtues are dispositions to make right choices, and that requires us not only to aim at the right goal, but get the means to that goal correct by prudent planning, decisions and commands. Prudence, in return, requires the moral virtues: correct reasoning about the means to be chosen must start from the goal to be achieved, and to that we are rightly disposed by moral virtues.[17]

For Aquinas, prudence is a subcategory, or special form, of practical reasoning: it is a virtue that involves reasoning rightly about things to be done; it requires good ends to distinguish itself from mere cunning; and it has an intimate role in moral deliberation – so much so that Aquinas listed prudence as both an intellectual and a moral virtue.[18] As with Aristotle's approach to practical wisdom and other virtues, Aquinas's understanding of prudence includes an element of desire by which a person wills the achievement of the good action that prudence discerns.[19] A further similarity with Aristotle is the ends-orientation that guides prudence as a form of practical reasoning, which "begins with the end and seeks the means of achieving it, moving from remote means to proximate and

[12] Aristotle, *Nicomachean ethics*, 169–70.
[13] Foot, "Virtues and vices," 105–106.
[14] Aquinas, *Summa theologica*, 377.
[15] Ibid., 376.
[16] Ibid., 377.
[17] Ibid., 243.
[18] Davies, *The thought of Thomas Aquinas*, 240–41.
[19] Aquinas, *Summa theologica*, 379; McInerny, "Ethics," 204–206.

arriving ultimately at what I can do here and now."[20] In short, Aquinas views prudence as the ability to deliberate about means and ends and put into practice the results of that deliberation.[21]

Aquinas's view of prudence as a form of practical reasoning is illustrated by the syllogistic manner in which practical reasoning progresses from a major premise (drawn from a principle), through a minor premise (based on an appraisal of one's particular circumstances in light of the principle), to a conclusion (a command of prudence) regarding what one ought to do.[22] Within this syllogistic paradigm, prudence entails apprehending the objective details of a situation, assessing those details in light of relevant moral principles, and responding to the situation on the basis of that assessment. The trajectory of prudence thereby moves from what one should do in general to what one should do in a particular set of circumstances. Moving from the former to the latter requires knowledge of the concrete details that define a given context of decision making. While the goal of virtue – that is, human flourishing – is innately known in general and in advance of particular circumstances, Aquinas maintains that the means of achieving this goal "are as various as the people and undertakings involved," and knowledge of those means is not innate.[23]

In Aquinas's philosophy there is an intimate relationship between prudence, conscience, and the ability to apprehend first principles of morality. Aquinas believed that human beings have a natural disposition to understand and assent to the first principles of morality.[24] These basic principles, such as "Good is to be done and evil avoided" or "Killing innocent people is wrong," are general and therefore ought to be specified as they are applied to the concrete circumstances of life. The rational ability to make this application – the minor premise in the preceding syllogism – is the ability of conscience.[25] Whereas the function of conscience is to apply moral knowledge to activity, the role of prudence is to execute the dictates of conscience.[26]

The relationship between prudence and the apprehension of reality receives considerable attention in the work of Josef Pieper, one of Aquinas's twentieth-century interpreters. Pieper shows how this relationship

[20] McInerny, "Ethics," 206–207.
[21] Aquinas, *Summa theologica*, 378.
[22] McInerny, "Ethics," 206.
[23] Aquinas, *Summa theologica*, 378–79.
[24] Davies, *The thought of Thomas Aquinas*, 233.
[25] Ibid., 234.
[26] Langston, *Conscience and other virtues*, 43.

is the result of Aquinas's understanding of the way human reason relates to human flourishing. To flourish, human beings need to live within the truth of the world as it exists, and this involves exercising reason in order to be open to and accept reality through the pursuit of truth.[27] As the ability to make right choices, prudence is preeminent among the virtues because it apprehends the reality on which our good depends. Writes Pieper: "Realization of the good presupposes that our actions are appropriate to the real situation, that is to the concrete realities which form the "environment" of a concrete human action; and that we therefore take this concrete reality seriously, with clear-eyed objectivity."[28] The interactive quality of prudence gives it a dual aspect of perception and expression as it both perceives the reality at hand and acts intentionally in response to it. This duality explains how imprudence can result from either thoughtlessness (lack of perception and deliberation) or irresoluteness (lack of action).[29]

In explicating Aquinas, Pieper makes a point of emphasizing how different Aquinas's notion of prudence can be from contemporary understandings of this term. To modern ears, *prudent* can connote a shrewdness regarding one's own self-interest. But this accent on self-interest was not present in the medieval understanding of prudence. Medieval culture had another term, *cunning* (in Latin, *astutia*), that represented false prudence, what Pieper describes as "the insidious and unobjective temperament of the intriguer who has regard only for 'tactics,' who can neither face things squarely nor act straightforwardly."[30] Cunning "blocks its subject from the truth of real things"[31] because of an anxious desire for self-preservation and an "immoderate straining for all the possessions which man thinks are needed to assure his own importance and status."[32]

As an illustration of the contrast between prudence and cunning, consider how a physician might discuss with a family the possibility of an autopsy after a patient of his died in the hospital after ten days of treatment. Consider further that the cause of death is uncertain and the physician is aware of circumstances that raise the possibility that a medical error caused or contributed to the patient's death. A prudent physician would recommend an autopsy as a source of information that might lead

[27] Pieper, *The four cardinal virtues*, 8–9.
[28] Ibid., 10.
[29] Ibid., 11–13.
[30] Ibid., 19–20.
[31] Ibid., 20.
[32] Ibid., 20–21.

to a better understanding of what happened, regardless of the implications of that understanding. A cunning physician might decide to remain silent about, or even discourage, an autopsy out of concern that its findings might implicate him in the death and thereby harm his perceived self-interests.

In the following summary Pieper describes the richness of Aquinas's understanding of prudence, as it places the moral agent *objectively* within a contextual reality that establishes the grounds for proper action and identifies the agent *subjectively* as one who desires to understand and act responsively on those grounds:

> Prudence, then, is the mold and mother of all virtues, the circumspect and resolute shaping power of our minds which transforms knowledge of reality into realization of the good. It holds within itself the humility of silent, that is to say, of unbiased perception; the trueness-to-being of memory; the art of receiving counsel; alert, composed readiness for the unexpected. Prudence means the studied seriousness and, as it were, the filter of deliberation, and at the same time the brave boldness to make final decisions. It means purity, straightforwardness, candor, and simplicity of character; it means standing superior to the utilitarian complexities of mere "tactics."[33]

Seen this way, prudence entails an openness to reality marked by a humility and a candor that stem from a desire to recognize and respond to the world as it is, rather than an attempt to impose our self-oriented desires and intentions onto the world.

II. FIVE CORE ELEMENTS OF PRACTICAL WISDOM

On the basis of the preceding discussion and in light of virtue ethics as considered in Chapter 2, practical wisdom can be seen as having multiple elements, all of which are relevant to the practice of medicine and ethics. Working within the virtue-based traditions elaborated by Aristotle and Aquinas and their interpreters, I would suggest that practical wisdom includes the following five core elements:

1. the pursuit of worthwhile ends (goals) derived from a concept of human flourishing;
2. an accurate perception of the concrete circumstances of a specific practical situation;

[33] Ibid., 22.

3. a commitment to moral virtues and principles that are interdependent and form an integrated moral framework;
4. deliberation that integrates ends (goals), concrete circumstances, and moral virtues and principles; and
5. the motivation to act in order to implement the conclusions reached by such deliberation.[34]

These core elements situate practical wisdom within a moral context established by the foundational beliefs and values that define our understanding of human flourishing and guide our commitment to moral virtues and principles. These elements also stand in close relation to conscience, for reasons that will be explored in the next chapter.

III. VIRTUES IN MEDICAL PRACTICE

Despite the challenges associated with virtue ethics discussed in Chapter 2, and even though principles tend to dominate contemporary bioethical discussions, there is an enduring awareness of the need for virtues in medical practice. That need is premised on distinctive features of medical practice that place an exceptionally high premium on professionals who are committed to fulfilling their fiduciary responsibilities to patients. As an illustration of this awareness, consider the way virtues are invoked in a position statement entitled "Patient–Physician Covenant," written by a group of physician-leaders concerned about the distorting effects of market forces and physician self-interest on medical practice. In this statement the authors assert that medicine "is a special kind of human activity – one that cannot be pursued effectively without the virtues of humility, honesty, intellectual integrity, compassion, and effacement of excessive self-interest."[35] The invocation of these virtues is clear and distinct, and the simplicity with which they are expressed reflects how recognizable they are believed to be.

Edmund Pellegrino argues that reliance on virtues is simply inescapable in medicine, since virtues inevitably pertain to any credible moral framework. In contemporary accounts of virtue ethics, he sees a reexamination and resurgence of classical and medieval concepts, as well as the recognition that virtues cannot be set aside by rights and principles, since

[34] For a previously published and substantially similar presentation of these five elements, see Lauris C. Kaldjian, "Teaching practical wisdom in medicine through clinical judgment, goals of care, and ethical reasoning," *Journal of Medical Ethics* 36 (2010): 558–62.

[35] Crawshaw et al., "Patient–physician covenant."

their moral effectiveness still depends on "the disposition and character traits of our fellow men and women."[36] He also believes that medical practice provides a context for virtues that has an advantage over the context of society generally speaking, since medicine can ground virtues in a specific framework of meaning based on the patient's good.[37]

In his work with David Thomasma on the virtues in medical practice, Pellegrino identified eight core virtues for medical practice: fidelity to trust, compassion, practical wisdom, justice, fortitude, temperance, integrity, and self-effacement.[38] Beauchamp and Childress offer an alternative set of core virtues in medicine that draw from an ethics of care based on the nature of relationships between patients and those who care for them. They propose one "fundamental" virtue, caring, accompanied by five supportive "focal" virtues (compassion, discernment, trustworthiness, integrity, and conscientiousness) that facilitate the development and expression of the virtue of caring.[39] Other virtues also exist – such as respectfulness, nonmalevolence, benevolence, and justice – but the six core virtues are thought to form the virtuous center of medical practice. In subsequent chapters I discuss the virtue of integrity and consider whether conscience should be seen as a virtue, but at this point it is sufficient to note that differences are evident among authors' selections of the virtues deemed most important for medicine.

Regarding the virtue of practical wisdom, Pellegrino and Thomasma describe it as "medicine's indispensable virtue" that disposes the physician to "attain the truth for the sake of action" and facilitates the coordinated expression of all other virtues in the process of achieving a right and good healing action for a patient.[40] They understand a *right* action as one that is determined by what is scientifically and technically appropriate, and a *good* action as one that is determined by what is in the patient's interests. This explains why they claim that the central cognitive activity of the physician, clinical judgment, requires practical wisdom,[41] for it joins the intellectual and moral aspects of the clinician's activity. Beauchamp and Childress acknowledge that what they call *discernment* is closely associated with practical wisdom, and they describe the practically wise person as one who knows which ends are valuable and how those ends can best be

36 Pellegrino, "The virtuous physician, and the ethics of medicine," 237.
37 Ibid., 238–47.
38 Pellegrino and Thomasma, *The virtues in medical practice.*
39 Beauchamp and Childress, *Principles of biomedical ethics*, 31–44.
40 Pellegrino and Thomasma, *The virtues in medical practice*, 84–86.
41 Ibid., 90.

realized in a particular context. Their remarks indicate appreciation for the wise person's ability to respond to the reality of the circumstances at hand, with sensitivity to the particularities of a given patient and his context that determines which principles of duty and virtues are most relevant. How principles and virtues are to be applied and balanced in a given case is a process that requires discernment, and it will show as much variability "as the ways in which devoted parents care for their children."[42]

IV. PRACTICAL WISDOM AND CLINICAL JUDGMENT

The claim by Pellegrino and Thomasma that clinical judgment requires practical wisdom warrants particular consideration, given what this claim implies for the relationship between the scientific and ethical aspects of clinical reasoning. As summarized in this chapter, practical wisdom is a teleological approach to decision making focused on ends, bounded by moral principles, informed by concrete circumstances, and driven by the right kinds of motivation. Assuming this account is valid, the claim that clinical judgment requires practical wisdom implies that clinical judgment is fundamentally a moral endeavor. To consider this implication, we should first clarify what clinical judgment means and consider whether its characteristics encompass the moral features that practical wisdom entails.

Some would say that clinical judgment is the principal inductive skill of the physician,[43] a skill by which she seeks to solve a medical problem through a process of data collection, the development and testing of hypotheses to explain the problem, and the formulation of recommendations for therapy based on those hypotheses,[44] a process that is sometimes referred to as "clinical reasoning."[45] Clinical judgment is defined in a more detailed way as the complete cognitive process by which a clinician "collects and interprets data; formulates a problem statement, confirms and refutes diagnostic hypotheses; considers, plans, and implements

[42] Beauchamp and Childress, *Principles of biomedical ethics*, 40.

[43] Elliott Sober, "The art and science of clinical judgment: an informational approach," in *Clinical judgment: a critical appraisal*, ed. H. Tristram Engelhardt, Stuart F. Spicker, and Bernard Towers (Dordrecht: Reidel, 1979), 32.

[44] Arthur S. Elstein, "Human factors in clinical judgment: discussion of Scriven's 'Clinical Judgment,'" in *Clinical judgment*, ed. Tristram Engelhardt et al., 20.

[45] Jerome P. Kassirer and Richard I. Kopelman, *Learning clinical reasoning* (Baltimore: Williams & Wilkins, 1991), 3.

possible diagnostic and therapeutic options, tests, and interventions; and evaluates likelihoods and outcomes."[46]

Despite definitional variations, there appears to be broad agreement that clinical judgment is an inductive and iterative skill involving the processing of information that transforms a host of data (from the history, physical exam, laboratory, and radiology) into a differential diagnosis (a manageable list of possible hypotheses that may explain a patient's problem) that are then sifted and further tested in an attempt to identify the most likely explanation for a malady and justify an approach to its treatment. Clinical judgment is commonly viewed as an explicitly cognitive process, and therefore open to elucidation by insights from cognitive science, decision theory, and computer science.[47] A less common view is that clinical judgment entails explicit *and* tacit elements, the latter of which are expressed not in conscious verbal descriptions about the mechanisms of clinical judgment, but through demonstration or "knowing-in-action."[48]

With respect to the relationship between ethics and science in medicine, it is important to consider whether the preceding descriptions of clinical judgment include a moral aspect. Such consideration encourages us to question whether clinical judgment is a cognitive skill that can be detached from ethical considerations or whether its demands are properly seen as both scientific and ethical. When reading accounts of clinical judgment or clinical reasoning that carry little in the way of ethical content, one presumes that ethical commitments are being taken for granted and left unstated rather than being detached or ignored. This seems to be the case in *Learning Clinical Reasoning*, by Jerome Kassirer and Richard Kopelman, which only goes so far as to acknowledge that choices about tests and treatments depend on assessments of the risks and benefits that are predicted to accrue from them.[49] These authors do not discuss the relevance of the ethical values and beliefs of patients or clinicians. Instead, they focus on decision thresholds based on the known efficacy, risks, and benefits of treatment, along with the physician's level of diagnostic confidence. By contrast, other writers on clinical judgment express recognition of the relation between ethical values and clinical concerns when they acknowledge, for instance, the ethical significance

46 Gilbert M. Goldman, "The tacit dimension of clinical judgment," *Yale Journal of Biology and Medicine* 63 (1990): 48.

47 Kassirer and Kopelman, *Learning clinical reasoning*, 3.

48 Goldman, "The tacit dimension of clinical judgment," 50.

49 Kassirer and Kopelman, *Learning clinical reasoning*, 5–6.

of making a wrong diagnosis[50] or the value-laden nature of clinical judgment due to the ethical dimension it inevitably entails.[51]

Even greater contrast is provided by Pellegrino, who claims that the ethical dimension of clinical judgment is its defining feature, since the moral dimension of medicine (a right and good healing action) gives clinical judgment its direction and purpose.[52] For Pellegrino, clinical judgment has multiple facets that are interwoven with ethical reasoning to determine whether or how tests and treatments will advance the interests of a particular patient. And he believes that this process of determination requires the virtue of practical wisdom, or prudence. Pellegrino's analysis offers a complex portrait of clinical judgment that entails genuine engagement between the physician and the patient in order to orient the outcome of all reasoning to the patient's good. He crystallizes the purpose of clinical judgment into three questions: What can be wrong? What can be done? What should be done? The third of these questions testifies to the ethical and patient-centered character of clinical judgment as it moves reasoning from the realm of scientific induction and deduction into the moral domain of the patient's good. When it is focused on the patient's good, clinical judgment has an ends-orientation that relates directly to practical wisdom.

Pellegrino's assessment helps us see that the relationship between clinical judgment and practical wisdom (in the medical context) is so close because both depend on the same primary moral ground – the good of the patient. Their differences at first glance seem obvious. Clinical judgment focuses on biomedical data, interpretation of data, hypotheses, probabilities, and treatments. Practical wisdom focuses on ends, principles, and motivations. But when clinical judgment is understood to be an inherently ethical endeavor focused on goals, its close relationship with practical wisdom warrants the conclusion that *clinical judgment simply is practical wisdom applied to the practice of medicine.* For clinical judgment is a matter of looking at the reality of the patient openly and truthfully and then deciding how best to respond, based on the ends in view, the means best suited to achieve those ends, and an appreciation for the moral principles and virtues necessary to guide and motivate diagnostic and therapeutic decisions.

[50] Sober, "The art and science of clinical judgment," 34–35.

[51] Michael Scriven, "Clinical judgment," in *Clinical judgment*, ed. Tristram Engelhardt et al., 12–13.

[52] Edmund D. Pellegrino, "The anatomy of clinical judgments: some notes on right reason and right action," in *Clinical judgment*, ed. Tristram Engelhardt et al., 169–94.

If this conclusion is correct, the way we understand, use, and teach clinical judgment can be enhanced if its relationship to practical wisdom is acknowledged. This would encourage us to make explicit the ethical purposes, values, and motivations that might otherwise be neglected in the process of exercising clinical judgment. Making these aspects of clinical judgment clear would help keep the ethical dimension of clinical judgment in the foreground as it is practiced and taught. Under pressure from a biomedical model that focuses primarily on diseases and diagnoses, clinical judgment that loses sight of its ethical dimension risks losing sight of patients as persons and the beliefs, values, and goals that define their lives.

There is another aspect of clinical judgment that reveals additional similarity with practical wisdom, and that is its dependence on training and practice. Those who write about clinical judgment describe it as a complex skill that cannot be acquired without such experience. Goldman notes the irreplaceable need for repetitive and supervised practice over years of training.[53] Sober likens the process of learning clinical judgment to that of learning to speak a language or play chess, both of which require that the learner participate in the process in order to understand it.[54] Pellegrino believes that the dialectical, ethical, and rhetorical aspects of clinical judgment reveal the need for education in the humanities as part of medical training, and he believes that this education is needed over the entire course of training, since the moral nature of many medical decisions becomes apparent to students only as they gain more direct clinical experience.[55]

V. SUMMARY

The demands of decision making in clinical medicine reflect a physician's need for practical wisdom, which involves knowing what ends or goals are worth pursuing and what means are most likely to achieve them. As understood in this chapter, practical wisdom entails an explicitly *ethical* dimension because it requires that we appreciate what is good for a patient as a person, not merely as a biological being.

Within the virtue tradition that traces back to Aristotle and Aquinas, practical wisdom is foremost among the cardinal virtues because it allows

[53] Goldman, "The tacit dimension of clinical judgment," 59.
[54] Sober, "The art and science of clinical judgment," 42–43.
[55] Pellegrino, "The anatomy of clinical judgments," 192.

those who possess it to respond realistically – in the sense of being true to reality – when faced with a challenging decision. Practical wisdom is the preeminent practical virtue because a proper understanding of when and how other virtues are to be expressed depends not merely on our good intentions but also on our ability to perceive and engage the objective features of a situation, as well as the moral values that pertain to it. Practical wisdom is distinguished from mere cleverness, in that the latter involves the pursuit of inappropriate ends or the willful neglect of one or more aspects of the circumstantial reality that ought, for the sake of truthfulness, to influence the pursuit of appropriate ends. Practical wisdom entails a humility that involves openness to the world as it is, in contrast to the tactical attempts of a cunning mind that attempts to impose its self-serving intentions onto the world. Drawing from the virtue-based traditions, practical wisdom can be understood to contain the five core elements enumerated in Section II of this chapter. These core elements show that practical wisdom depends on the foundational beliefs and values that define our understanding of human flourishing and guide our commitment to moral virtues and principles. As a result, these elements also invite consideration of the relationship between practical wisdom and conscience, which will be explored in the next chapter.

In the context of medicine, practical wisdom can be compared to clinical judgment. Both practical wisdom and clinical judgment are guided by ends or goals that arise from the same moral ground – the good of the patient. And though their commonly articulated features might seem to imply that they are different, an alternative view would hold that clinical judgment, when properly understood, is simply practical wisdom as it is manifested in the context of medicine. For clinical judgment is a matter of looking at the patient's situation openly and truthfully and then deciding how best to respond to it, given the goals to be pursued, the means best suited to achieve those goals, and an appreciation for the moral considerations necessary to guide and motivate decision making. Clinical judgment qualifies as practical wisdom when its ethical purposes – values, motivations, and goals of care – are made explicit and incorporated. Understanding clinical judgment this way helps remind physicians that clinical decision making is a moral process, and should always be treated as such, because it is concerned with patients as persons who have beliefs, values, and goals that must be respected.

A narrower biomedical view of clinical judgment may at times appear to be sufficient when clinical attention is concentrated on the technicalities of diseases, diagnoses, and possible treatments. But a more complete perspective of clinical judgment that includes the ethical dimension should never be lost from view. If that dimension is neglected, there is a risk that we will loosen our grip on the continuous need to engage the patient as a person by informing, listening, and sharing the process of decision making. The more we allow patient-centered ethical concerns to facilitate genuine dialogue with patients, the less likely it is that "clinical judgment" will merely represent "a clinician's judgment."

4

Conscience and Its Relation to Practical Wisdom

In the preceding chapter it was noted that the five core elements of practical wisdom depend on foundational beliefs and values that determine our understanding of human flourishing and guide our commitment to moral virtues and principles. It was also suggested that these elements invite consideration of the relationship between practical wisdom and conscience. This relationship will be discussed at the end of this chapter. But first, it is important to review past and present conceptions of conscience and discuss how they are related to both reason and religious faith.

I. HISTORICAL PERSPECTIVES ON CONSCIENCE

The concept of *conscience* has a complex history, and an appreciation of its origins and transformations over the past two thousand years facilitates a deeper understanding of the diverse ways in which conscience has been conceived. To the extent that current conceptions of conscience have been influenced by this history, a look to the past helps clarify the diverse assessments of conscience one finds in contemporary discussions. To portray something of this history, I will sketch some of the major contributions to the concept of conscience as they have come to us through Christian traditions, and I will then refer to some philosophical and psychological developments that followed these Christian renditions. This sketch is selective and intended to provide an introduction to the range of past conceptions and their developments over time.[1]

[1] For an extended analysis of the history of conscience, see Langston, *Conscience and other virtues*.

According to the analysis of C. A. Pierce, the notion of conscience emerged in the Greek world only after the collapse of the city-state, due to the loss of the integration of politics and ethics and the subsequent absence of an external moral authority to direct individual conduct. As a consequence of this ethical-political transformation, people "fell back on the internal chastisement of conscience as the only authority."[2] By the first century B.C., the idea of conscience as a moral notion had come into use in the Greek world, even though it was neither a developed nor a uniform concept.[3] But a major shift came in the Christian era by way of the apostle Paul, who attributed to conscience what Maurer describes as the "central self-consciousness of knowing and acting man."[4] The reliance on the individual authority of conscience was particularly evident in a dispute among Christians in first-century Corinth, which forced Paul to use the Greco-Roman notion of conscience in the context of early Christian culture.[5] Mature Christians in Corinth were eating food that had been sacrificed to idols and were rightly claiming to have a clear conscience about doing so. However, less mature Christians, who still believed eating food that had been sacrificed to idols was wrong, were emboldened to follow the example of the mature Christians and were thereby compromising themselves by doing what they believed was wrong. Paul was compelled to admonish mature Christians to avoid using their freedom in such a way as to cause less mature Christians to act against their consciences.[6]

In his admonition, Paul borrowed the existing Greek idea of conscience (in Greek, *syneidesis*), even though he perceived its limitations as a negative moral norm. The Greek notion of conscience that Paul introduced into Christian thought involved the pain a person experiences after doing what is wrong, a pain that arises because "man is by nature so constituted that, if he oversteps the moral limits of his nature he will normally feel pain – the pain called *syneidesis*."[7] On this view, conscience applies to actions that are bad and in the past, and conscience has an authority that is limited to the person whose action and conscience are at issue.[8]

[2] C. A. Pierce, *Conscience in the New Testament* (London: SCM Press, 1955), 76.

[3] Christian Maurer, "† σύνοιδα, † συνείδησις," in *Theological dictionary of the New Testament*, ed. Gerhard Kittel and Gerhard Friedrich (Grand Rapids, MI: Eerdmans, 1971), 906–909.

[4] Ibid., 917.

[5] Pierce, *Conscience in the New Testament.*

[6] I Corinthians 8. *Bible*, New International Version (Grand Rapids, MI: Zondervan, 1996).

[7] Pierce, *Conscience in the New Testament*, 50.

[8] Ibid., 45.

In his admonition, Paul endeavored to show that the positive claims of Christian love were greater than the negative claims of a free conscience: "'Everything is permissible' – but not everything is beneficial. 'Everything is permissible' – but not everything is constructive. Nobody should seek his own good, but the good of others."[9] In summary, Pierce detects three characteristics of conscience in the New Testament. It is a universal phenomenon among humans, it manifests as a painful reaction against infringements on human nature, and it is limited by human fallibility and the susceptibility to misinformation.[10] This conscience, says Pierce,

> is the reaction of the whole man to his own wrong acts. It is a moral reflex action, parallel, but also akin, to those reactions that make a man drop a red hot poker or spew out a poison, long before conscious reasoning has been brought to bear on those objects. The absolute pitch of the trained musician is likewise akin to the moral 'absolute pitch' of the trained Christian: the wrong note – be it ever so little wrong – causes immediate pain.[11]

While Pierce discerns a predominantly retrospective character of conscience in the New Testament,[12] D'Arcy views Paul as introducing both a retrospective and a prospective aspect of conscience. On this view, conscience has not only a judgmental (judicial) role that operates after an action has occurred, but also a directive (legislative) role that operates beforehand while an action is contemplated. D'Arcy sees the prospective aspect and fallibility of conscience as two features that distinguish Paul's concept of conscience from the Greco-Roman understanding that preceded it.[13]

Within the Roman Catholic tradition, the work of Thomas Aquinas (1225–74) has exerted a seminal influence on the understanding of conscience. Aquinas believed that conscience was "the activity of consciously applying our knowledge to what we do: witnessing to what we do and don't do, legislating about what we should and shouldn't do, and defending or accusing us when we have or haven't done well."[14] On this view, conscience has both prospective and retrospective roles, and its fundamental character is derived from practical reason – that is, from the ability to apply knowledge to action. Rather than being some sort of special faculty or

9 I Corinthians 10:23–24.

10 Pierce, *Conscience in the New Testament*, 108, 13.

11 Ibid., 113.

12 Ibid., 108.

13 Eric D'Arcy, *Conscience and its right to freedom* (New York: Sheed and Ward, 1961), 11–12.

14 Aquinas, *Summa theologica*, 124.

innate sense of moral perception, conscience is "a judgment of ordinary human reason brought to bear on a moral issue,"[15] and it functions in a syllogistic fashion, as follows:

1. We grasp by what he calls *synderesis* (which is not to be confused with *syneidesis*) self-evident, basic moral principles (major premise);
2. We make judgments about an action within a given set of circumstances (minor premise);
3. We draw conclusions about the goodness or badness of that action (conclusion).[16]

Seen this way, conscience is a matter of applying basic moral principles (e.g., "Murdering is bad") to specific actions and circumstances ("This action is an instance of murder in this circumstance") to reach a practical conclusion ("This action should not be done in this circumstance").[17]

For Aquinas, conscience produces judgments about what is right and wrong after everything relevant has been taken into consideration. Conscience therefore represents a person's "last, best judgment that a course of action is or is not morally correct."[18] For Aquinas and many others, this explains why there is no higher decision-making standard against which to compare the conclusions of conscience. If there were any such standards and if those standards were known to the individual, they would already have been incorporated into the individual's considerations. As will be discussed in the next chapter, this is why Aquinas and others have believed that one ought always to follow the conclusions of conscience even if one's conscience happens to be, from some other perspective, mistaken. Simply put, conscience represents the culmination of an individual's most informed and best efforts in moral decision making. If there is a course of action that is morally superior to what an individual's conscience has determined, by definition the individual is not in a position to recognize that morally superior action since her conscience has not already identified it. Of course, with further

[15] Eric D'Arcy, "Conscience," *Journal of Medical Ethics* 3 (1977): 98–99.

[16] Davies, *The thought of Thomas Aquinas*, 235.

[17] Curran observes that this syllogistic understanding of conscience has had an enduring presence in the Catholic tradition. See Charles E. Curran, "Conscience in the light of the Catholic moral tradition," in *Conscience*, ed. Charles E. Curran (Mahwah, NJ: Paulist Press, 2004), 7–8.

[18] Germain Grisez and Russell Shaw, "Conscience: knowledge of moral truth," in *Conscience*, ed. Curran, 43.

information and reasoning, the conclusion of an individual's conscience may be changed. Such changes indicate the importance of achieving a properly informed conscience.

In contrast to Aquinas, Martin Luther (1483–1546) represents what Langston calls a "Protestant turn" in the focus of conscience, a turn from actions to persons.[19] While Luther did not completely abandon the traditional relationship between conscience and practical reason, he viewed the primary role of conscience as a matter of self-judgment, of judging the whole of one's own person. The unintended consequence of this turn, according to Langston, is that it facilitated movement toward a conception of conscience as an entity independent of reason. "Once conscience is no longer thought of as a part of a process (of practical reason) and is viewed as something like a judge of the whole person, the way is prepared for conceiving of conscience as an independent entity."[20] In a similar assessment, Zachman observes that although Luther followed Aquinas in accepting that conscience works by reason according to the logic of a practical syllogism whereby the moral value of individual actions are judged,[21] he departed from Aquinas in maintaining that "the proper domain of the conscience lies in placing the person before the judgment seat of God on the basis of works, and of giving forth a judgment that makes us either accused or saved before God."[22] Understood within a Lutheran theological framework that places faith prior to works, the result of the proper work of conscience is to show the individual that he cannot have a good conscience – cannot be or do good – without God's gracious gift of forgiveness.[23] Thus construed, a good conscience is given to the Christian not as a consequence of doing good, but from a willingness to accept God's justifying forgiveness (salvation). Subsequent to this acceptance, the Christian, according to Luther, can act with a conscience that is "good" by virtue of God's grace, not because of human effort or accomplishment.

Like Luther, John Calvin (1509–64) viewed the primary work of conscience as providing the means for humans to perceive the divine judgment of their sins:

[19] Langston, *Conscience and other virtues*, 77.

[20] Ibid.

[21] Randall C. Zachman, *The assurance of faith: conscience in the theology of Martin Luther and John Calvin* (Louisville: Westminster John Knox Press, 2005), 28.

[22] Ibid., 24.

[23] Paul Althaus, *The ethics of Martin Luther* (Philadelphia: Fortress Press, 1972), 4–6.

> [W]hen [humans] have a sense of divine judgment, as a witness joined to them, which does not allow them to hide their sins from being accused before the Judge's tribunal, this sense is called "conscience." For it is a certain mean between God and man, because it does not allow man to suppress within himself what he knows, but pursues him to the point of convicting him.[24]

For Calvin, God speaks to humans through their consciences and thereby brings them to the same judgment of themselves that God has.[25] On this understanding, the voice of conscience is the voice of God.

In the history of the concept of conscience, Joseph Butler (1692–1752) is known for treating conscience as if it were a "moral sense,"[26] imbued with the capacity to perceive right and wrong akin to the immediacy by which the sense of taste perceives sweet and sour. An influential Anglican clergyman, Butler believed that conscience was implanted by God in humans to represent God's commands. As such, conscience was seen as infallible and having the purpose of judging persons and their actions.[27] Because of his view of conscience as a moral sense organ, Butler is credited as the person perhaps most responsible for modern views that conceive of conscience as a distinct faculty that is independent of reason.[28] This attribution is understandable in light of the second of Butler's Five Sermons,[29] in which he refers to conscience as a "faculty" consisting of a "particular kind of reflection"[30] that, along with cool self-love, stands in contrast to the passions that otherwise compel human behavior. The immediacy of this faculty of conscience is such that it "pronounces determinately some actions to be in themselves just, right, good; others to be in themselves evil, wrong, unjust, which, without being consulted, without being advised with, magisterially exerts itself, and approves or condemns him the doer of them accordingly."[31] For Butler, the faculty of conscience constitutes the basis of human moral agency,[32] and in its surveying, approving, and disapproving it has a "sacred" authority "to be our proper

[24] John Calvin, *Institutes of the Christian religion*, ed. John T. McNeill (Philadelphia: Westminster Press, 1960), 848.
[25] Zachman, *The assurance of faith*, 100.
[26] Davies, *The thought of Thomas Aquinas*, 235.
[27] Langston, *Conscience and other virtues*, 81–82.
[28] Ibid., 80.
[29] Joseph Butler, *Five sermons* (Indianapolis: Hackett, 1983).
[30] Ibid., 35.
[31] Ibid., 37.
[32] Ibid.

governor, to direct and regulate all under principles, passions, and motives of action."[33]

Despite these references to conscience as a faculty, it should be noted that Butler also referred to conscience as a kind of reflection, implying that he also saw reason as being active in the function of conscience. Accordingly, some would argue that Butler affirmed both "moral reason" and "moral sense" and that his depiction of conscience is that of a faculty of genuine discrimination, reflection, and judgment.[34] This broader view of conscience is illustrated by Butler's reference (in *A Dissertation upon the Nature of Virtue*) to "a moral faculty, whether called conscience, moral reason, moral sense, or divine reason; whether considered as a sentiment of the understanding or as a perception of the heart, or, which seems the truth, as including both."[35] In any case, Butler's influence on the conceptualization of conscience as a distinct faculty has been substantial, even if we are left to wonder whether all of his interpreters have appreciated the full nuance of his assessment of the role reason plays in conscience.

Immanuel Kant (1724–1804) had a view of conscience similar to that of Butler. For Kant, conscience was "something like a universal moral judge" and therefore relevant not only to the person whose conscience is in view, but to all moral agents who stand in relation to that person.[36] In his *Lectures on Ethics*, Kant describes conscience as "not a mere faculty, but an instinct" which passes judgment that "is not logical, but judicial."[37] Conscience, for Kant, functions like a judge who not only forms a judgment, but also passes judgment and must either condemn or acquit. "If our conscience were merely an impulse to form a judgment, it would be, like other faculties of which we are possessed . . . a faculty of knowledge."[38] Using the analogy of a court of law, Kant illustrates the function of conscience in this way:

> We find in our hearts a prosecutor, for whom there would be no place unless there were also a law. This law, which is based on reason and not on sentiment, is incorruptible and incontestably just and pure; it is the moral law, established as the holy and inviolable law of humanity. Beside these there is equally an advocate within us, called Self-love, who brings forward many an

33 Ibid., 40.

34 Brian Hebblethwaite, *Ethics and religion in a pluralistic age* (Edinburgh: T. & T. Clark, 1997), 40.

35 Butler, *Five sermons*, 69.

36 Langston, *Conscience and other virtues*, 83.

37 Immanuel Kant, *Lectures on ethics* (Indianapolis: Hackett, 1963), 129.

38 Ibid.

> argument in our defence, and whose pleas the prosecutor in his turn endeavours to refute. Lastly we find a judge within us who either condemns or acquits. It is impossible to blind his judgment. To refuse to appear before the bar of conscience is easier. Once we appear, the judge pronounces impartially, and his verdict falls normally upon the side of truth. If not, it must be because he judges by false principles of morality.[39]

Over time, conceptualizations of conscience emerged that distinguished it from practical reason, causing some interpreters to view conscience as an independent faculty that is "infallible, directive, and punitive, and the guarantor of morality."[40] Such a portrayal became the standard view of the nineteenth and early twentieth centuries, including the Freudian psychological assessment that conscience is a punishing judge linked (but not identified) with the superego.[41]

II. CONTEMPORARY CONCEPTIONS AND ASSESSMENTS OF CONSCIENCE

As shown by these historical examples, conscience has been given various meanings over the past two thousand years. This variability persists into modern times, and its contrasting conceptions have been described, in rapid-fire fashion, as follows:

> It has been said of conscience that it is fallible (Broad), that it is infallible (Butler); that its ultimate basis is emotional (Mill), that its ultimate source is rational (Rashdall); that it is the voice of God (Hartmann), or the voice of custom (Paulsen); that it is merely advisory (Nowell-Smith), that it is a command internally imposed (Mayo); that it is conscious (Butler), that it is unconscious (Freud); that it is a faculty (Butler), that it is not (any contemporary philosopher); that it is the disposition to have certain beliefs, emotions, and conations which, when operative, issue in conscientious actions (Broad), and that it *is* conscientious action (Ryle).[42]

Given such diversity, it might be tempting to conclude that a concept that is the object of so much dispute must be inherently faulty – perhaps because its reach exceeds its ability to grasp such an expansive, nuanced, and multifaceted subject. Alternatively, however, it might be suggested that the enduring intellectual, practical, and political interest in conscience

39 Ibid., 132.

40 Langston, *Conscience and other virtues*, 84.

41 Ibid., 91.

42 Bernard Wand, "The content and function of conscience," in *Conscience*, ed. John Donnelly and Leonard Lyons (Staten Island, NY: Alba House, 1973), 140–41.

indicates that, whatever the challenges, the notion of conscience continues to capture aspects of moral experience that remain broadly meaningful and highly significant. These challenges are not to be taken lightly, especially since some modern critics are ready to dismiss the notion of conscience entirely.[43] Nevertheless, we can agree with Langston and others who defend the continued use of the concept if we believe that it helps us focus on core aspects of the moral life, even if we lack consensus on how it should be interpreted, where its boundaries should be drawn, and what the political implications of its freedom should be. To this end, I believe that the challenges posed by the diverse conceptions of conscience should encourage two responses. First, and practically speaking, when we engage in discussions about conscience, we should explain to each other what we mean by conscience so that we do not mistakenly presume a shared understanding of its nature and significance. Second, we should continue to consider which conceptions of conscience appear to most effectively capture the moral, mental, and behavioral features perceived as being most relevant to the contexts in which conscience is discussed. By examining how contemporary writers conceive of conscience, we may determine which of its attributes are most central and, thereby, gain a clearer understanding of the role conscience should play in discussions about the practice of medicine and ethics.

Within the contemporary literature on conscience, there continue to be those who describe conscience as a manifestation of practical reason, as Aquinas and others have done previously. Dinneen, for instance, holds that conscience is "the exercise of practical reason on matters of moral values," since moral values and laws "need to be applied to particular acts by particular persons.[44] Similarly, D'Arcy describes conscience as being a matter of reasoned judgment, not some sort of intellectual or emotional "allergic reaction" to things perceived to be morally objectionable. Conscience, he writes, "is simply *myself*, making reasoned judgments about moral questions"; and one uses the same mental abilities when making moral judgments as when making judgments about anything else.[45]

In addition to the reasoning function of conscience, other writers add the notion of a sanction that attaches to its conclusions. According to

[43] Langston, *Conscience and other virtues*, 100, 107.

[44] John A. Dinneen, "Freedom of conscience in philosophical perspective," in *Conscience: its freedom and limitations*, ed. William C. Bier (New York: Fordham University Press, 1971), 103.

[45] D'Arcy, "Conscience."

Childress, for example, conscience functions as a sanction that arises from a person's reflection on, and consciousness of, her own actions in relation to her own standards of judgment; a reasoned judgment of rightness or wrongness occurs, and then this consciousness arises, whether retrospectively or prospectively.[46] With his colleague Beauchamp, he emphasizes the interweaving roles of reason, reflection, and sanction by describing conscience as both "a form of self-reflection on, and judgment about, whether one's acts are obligatory or prohibited, right or wrong, good or bad" and "an internal sanction that comes into play through critical reflection" that may manifest as feelings of remorse, guilt, or shame when an individual recognizes his committed acts as wrong.[47] Comparing Childress's view with that of Dinneen or D'Arcy, we can see a contrast between what we may call a two-dimensional (cognitive and emotive) and a one-dimensional (cognitive) characterization of conscience.

The significance of multidimensionality is seen even more clearly in the three-dimensional characterization of conscience provided by C. D. Broad, whose analysis has been influential. On his account, conscience consists of three related moral capacities: moral cognition, morally directed emotion, and moral motivation (the last being referred to as a conative disposition). To say that a person has a conscience is to assert the following three propositions: "(1) That he has and exercises the cognitive power of reflecting on his own past and future actions, and considering whether they are right or wrong; of reflecting on his own motives, intentions, emotions, disposition, and character, and considering whether they are morally good or bad; and of reflecting on the relative moral value of various alternative ideals of character and conduct. (2) That he has and exercises the emotional disposition to feel certain peculiar emotions, such as remorse, feeling of guilt, moral approval, etc., towards himself and his own actions, dispositions, etc., in respect of the moral characteristics which he believes these to have. (3) That he has and exercises the conative disposition to seek what he believes to be good and to shun what he believes to be bad, as such, and to do what he believes to be right and avoid what he believes to be wrong, as such."[48]

Given the extent to which a three-dimensional moral capacity involving reason, emotion, and motivation captures aspects of historical renditions

[46] James F. Childress, "Appeals to conscience," *Ethics* 89 (1979): 315–35.

[47] Beauchamp and Childress, *Principles of biomedical ethics*, 44.

[48] C. D. Broad, "Conscience and conscientious action," in *Conscience*, ed. Donnelly and Lyons, 8.

of conscience as well as its common usage, it is not surprising to see how Broad's assessment echoes in other writers. Sidney Callahan describes conscience as "a personal, self-conscious activity, integrating reason, emotion, and will in self-committed decision about right and wrong, good and evil."[49] Daniel Sulmasy maintains that conscience is an activity that "unifies the cognitive, conative, and emotional aspects of the moral life" and arises from a fundamental commitment to be moral.[50] Pellegrino refers to conscience as that which motivates the moral agent to follow the judgments of practical reason (deduced from natural law) or suffer the pangs of guilt, remorse, and shame.[51] Langston endorses Broad's conceptualization outright, placing special emphasis on how it represents conscience as a "relational entity" (as opposed to a "substantial entity," or faculty).[52]

A related example of a multidimensional view of conscience is offered by A. Campbell Garnett, for whom conscience has "both a cognitive and an emotive or motivational element."[53] The cognitive aspect judges what is morally right or wrong, while the emotive aspect provides emotions of approval or disapproval of actions that are judged right or wrong. Garnett's special concern is to draw attention to the capacity of the emotive part of conscience to function uncritically. "Because of this uncritical emotive reaction conscience all too frequently moves people to approve or disapprove actions and rules concerning which adequate reflection would lead to a very different verdict, and sometimes it afflicts people with a quite irrational sense of guilt."[54] Garnett criticizes reliance on conscience when it is uncritical or unreflective, and he equates the uncritical conscience with Butler's view, which he calls the "traditional" conscience, because it adopts traditional beliefs without first subjecting them to critical reevaluation.

A contrasting view is offered by Peter Fuss. Although multidimensional and relational, his interpretation of conscience omits the cognitive aspect of moral reasoning. Fuss omits this aspect because he believes that

[49] Sidney Callahan, *In good conscience: reason and emotion in moral decision making* (New York: HarperCollins, 1991), 14.

[50] Daniel P. Sulmasy, "What is conscience and why is respect for it so important?" *Theoretical Medicine and Bioethics* 29 (2008): 138.

[51] Edmund D. Pellegrino, "The physician's conscience, conscience clauses, and religious belief: a Catholic perspective," *Fordham Urban Law Journal* 30 (2002): 226–27.

[52] Langston, *Conscience and other virtues*, 126–27.

[53] A. Campbell Garnett, "Conscience and conscientiousness," in *Moral concepts*, ed. Joel Feinberg (Oxford: Oxford University Press, 1982), 81.

[54] Ibid., 82.

conscience has no intrinsic content, since its function is to motivate us to make our actions consistent with our moral knowledge and beliefs, *whatever* our moral knowledge and beliefs may be. Seen this way, conscience is literally *acting with knowledge* (*con-scientia*), such that we are disposed "to do what we think."[55] For Fuss, the distinctive role of conscience in the moral life is not to determine what we should do, but to ensure that once we reach our conclusions our actions will be consistent with our beliefs. He maintains that conscience

> does this by constituting a certain relation between the individual's moral knowledge or belief and his action. Namely, it establishes in the moral agent a felt need or disposition to act in accordance with his knowledge or belief, giving him a sense of personal integrity when he does so as best he can, and a corresponding sense of inner failure, frustration, or guilt when, through some fault of his own, he fails to do so.[56]

The demand for coherence between moral belief and action that Fuss ascribes to conscience resonates with the belief that whenever we accept a moral truth, we are recognizing that there is a necessary connection between *accepting* a moral truth and *acting* on the knowledge communicated by that truth. As Austin Duncan-Jones puts it, "[I]f I accept a moral truth and fail to act on it, I am not [doing all that my belief in the proposition demands]: and my not doing so appears almost as a kind of logical absurdity – as though I accepted a proposition and denied its self-evident implications."[57] Martin McGuire speaks similarly when claiming that "the force and function of a man's conscience is to encourage him to *follow* his judgment,"[58] an emphasis found also in Childress, who remarks that conscience "demands consistency between belief and action."[59]

Because accepting something to be morally true may be construed as a subjective affirmation rather than an objective claim, some commentators have addressed the relationship between conscience and truth and proposed a mediating role for conscience between subjective and objective perspectives regarding truth. Germain Grisez and Russell Shaw, for instance, believe that conscience "is one's awareness of moral truth – of that which is truly right and good to do" and that this awareness arises in response to

55 Peter Fuss, "Conscience," in *Conscience*, ed. Donnelly and Lyons, 47.

56 Ibid., 43.

57 Austin Duncan-Jones, "The notion of conscience," in *Conscience*, ed. Donnelly and Lyons, 126–27.

58 Martin C. McGuire, "On conscience," in *Conscience*, ed. Donnelly and Lyons, 155.

59 James Childress, "Conscience and conscientious actions in the context of MCOs," *Kennedy Institute of Ethics Journal* 7 (1997): 404.

our encounter with reality and the alternatives within that reality that present choices that allow us to fulfill our moral responsibilities.[60] Joseph Ratzinger (Pope Emeritus Benedict XVI) portrays conscience as directly related to, and dependent on, objective moral truth, and he dismisses the idea that conscience is merely a self-conscious, subjective certainty of one's moral behavior. He affirms Newman's claim that the truth on which conscience depends establishes the connection between the authority of conscience and its subjectivity, since conscience signifies "the voice of truth in the subject himself."[61] This connection explains why Ratzinger believes that conscience is properly understood as "co-knowing" with the truth and is not to be equated with personal preference or social consensus.[62] Ratzinger discerns this co-knowledge – this endowed ability that causes us to resonate with some things and clash with others – in Plato's concept of *anamnesis*, St. Paul's description of the law written on the heart, and Aquinas's notion of *synderesis* (our grasp of self-evident, basic moral principles).[63] In the next chapter's discussion of the authority and fallibility of conscience, I will return to questions regarding subjective and objective perspectives of truth.

III. CONSCIENCE AND REASON

Because of the irreplaceable role that reason plays in professional ethics and public policy, it is important to appreciate how significant it is that some conceptions of conscience portray it as intimately related to the ability to reason. For if conscience is not seen as part of our rational capacity – and is instead conceived of as some kind of private, inaccessible domain of discernment – then its relevance to professional and public spheres will be questionable. However, if conscience is believed to be part of reason, then its function and conclusions should be intelligible to other persons and relevant to moral deliberations in professional and public spheres. As already noted, a reason-based account of conscience is found in Aquinas, who considered it to be an expression of practical reason by which we make judgments when we are faced with moral questions and decisions. Similar accounts are found in modern discussions that claim the function of conscience is, in whole or in part, the application of

[60] Grisez and Shaw, "Conscience: knowledge of moral truth," 41.
[61] Joseph Ratzinger, *On conscience* (San Francisco: Ignatius Press, 2007), 25.
[62] Ibid., 27–28.
[63] Ibid., 30–32.

our general cognitive powers to concerns that are moral,[64] the means by which humans apply general moral values and laws to the particularities of concrete situations,[65] or "the human mind making moral judgments about a practical course of action."[66] According to these accounts, conscience is part of reason and, therefore, it is open to interpersonal criticism and the possibility of revision.

The rational character of conscience can be seen clearly in Aquinas's belief that conscience reasons along the lines of a syllogism – beginning with our understanding of self-evident and basic moral principles, proceeding to judgments about concrete circumstances and actions, and ending with conclusions about the goodness or badness of an action.[67] This syllogistic conception of conscience was also part of Luther's understanding.[68] For both Aquinas and Luther, the major premises upon which conscience depends are always true. But the usefulness of these truths is limited by their exceedingly general character, composed as they are of commonly affirmed moral beliefs such as "All sin is to be avoided" or "Everything good is to be done."[69] The challenge, of course, comes in determining the validity of the minor premises whose content derives from rational assessments of the moral status of a specific action within a concrete set of circumstances (e.g., "To strike down this man *in this situation* would be an act of self-defense, not murder").

Reliance on self-evident, basic moral truths indicates the important role played by natural law in conceptions of conscience in the work of Aquinas, Luther, and others in the Christian tradition. Such authors assume that a generally shared attribute of adult human beings is the ability to comprehend an objective moral order in the world – an order that makes fundamental moral claims on all human beings, such as prohibitions against murder, stealing, and lying. This comprehension of moral truth is believed to be a general human characteristic, whether a person believes in God or not. The role of natural law in the function of conscience is particularly strong in Catholic conceptions, as seen in Dolan's summary statement that conscience "is simply the extension or

64 D'Arcy, "Conscience."
65 Dinneen, "Freedom of conscience in philosophical perspective," 103.
66 John J. Hardt, "The conscience debate: resources for rapprochement from the problem's perceived source," *Theoretical Medicine and Bioethics* 29 (2008): 151–60.
67 Davies, *The thought of Thomas Aquinas*, 235.
68 Zachman, *The assurance of faith*, 24–25.
69 Ibid.

application of [the] natural law to a particular act."[70] (For completeness, it should be noted that the Catholic tradition also holds that, in the life of a Christian, conscience is influenced by faith, since faith informs reason through gifts – such as wisdom – imparted by the Holy Spirit that guide the discernment of conscience.)[71]

A definitive role for reason in the function of conscience can also be seen in some philosophical conceptions, including those that distinguish between an instinctive (traditional) conscience and a critical (reflective) one. Garnett provides such an example. He perceives in conscience both emotive and cognitive elements, and believes that conscience is merely traditional when the emotive element functions apart from the cognitive. By contrast, conscience is critical when it causes us to think for ourselves about what we really ought to do, by fixing our moral eyes firmly on the impact our actions have, for better or worse, on the persons around us. This critical moral reflection, he maintains, is the root of conscience.[72] David Little offers a similar perspective when he interprets both Aquinas and Kant as portraying conscience as fundamentally about giving reasons for actions, especially actions that affect other human beings.[73] The reflective aspect of conscience to which writers refer may be either prospective or retrospective, depending on whether it precedes or follows an act of moral judgment.

Within traditions that conceive of conscience as part of human reason, attention is also given to how reason relates to the will. For Aquinas, there is a lively interdependence between these two entities, because the "will can only be drawn to what reason perceives to be good" and, conversely, reasoning "depends on our willing the right goal."[74] Sulmasy echoes this assessment when stating that conscience involves the "conjunction of will and judgment."[75] The integration of reason and will in the function of conscience can also be detected in philosophical assessments recognizing the inseparability of moral belief and moral action that is implied when a moral claim is accepted as true. Such assessments claim that accepting a moral truth without acting on it is almost logically absurd, for doing

70 Joseph V. Dolan, "Conscience in the Catholic theological tradition," in *Conscience*, ed. Bier, 11.

71 Curran, "Conscience in the light of the Catholic moral tradition," 16.

72 Garnett, "Conscience and conscientiousness," 84–85.

73 David Little, "A view of conscience within the Protestant theological tradition," in *Conscience*, ed. Bier, 22–23.

74 Aquinas, *Summa theologica*, 196.

75 Sulmasy, "What is conscience and why is respect for it so important?" 138.

so would be to accept a proposition without accepting its self-evident implications.[76] By integrating reason and will, conscience encompasses a domain of beliefs – moral convictions – that are distinguished from other kinds of beliefs by virtue of their implications for action. For such beliefs, the will toward action is inseparable from the conclusions of reason. Of note, the relationship between will and reason in conscience parallels the relationship between motivation and deliberation in practical wisdom described in Chapter 3.

IV. CONSCIENCE AND RELIGIOUS FAITH

Though conscience can be conceived in rational terms that need not depend on religious faith, its history – as illustrated in the thought of Luther, Calvin, and Butler – shows how it has often been embedded in, and in vital ways dependent on, an explicitly religious foundation, especially in the Christian traditions. If we appreciate how some people may conceive of conscience in relation to religious faith, we will be more likely to understand the breadth and depth of its potential implications in contexts where religious faith is expressed, assumed, or accepted.

The relationship between religious faith and conscience is perhaps most palpable in the Protestant Christian traditions represented by Luther and Calvin. For Luther, conscience was a universal human attribute that functioned fundamentally as an indicator of a person's relationship with God, reflecting either a state of guilt (causing a bad conscience) or a state of forgiveness (resulting in a good conscience). Consistent with Luther's belief that forgiveness (salvation) is independent of human effort, a good conscience cannot be achieved by good deeds; rather, a good conscience is a gift from God that comes through the acceptance of the sin-canceling (justifying) work of Jesus Christ, by which the conscience is made good and becomes the source (not the product) of human efforts to do good works.[77] Calvin also understood conscience as a universal human attribute that indicates to a person that he is either guilty or forgiven before God. This universal work of conscience is intimately related to the ability to apprehend fundamental aspects of morality (natural law), but the key function of conscience for Calvin was to provide people knowledge of their sin that renders them inexcusable before God. As Calvin stated, "This would not be a bad definition: natural law is that apprehension of

[76] Duncan-Jones, "The notion of conscience," 126.
[77] Althaus, *The ethics of Martin Luther*, 4–6.

the conscience which distinguishes sufficiently between just and unjust, and which deprives men of the excuse of ignorance, while it proves them guilty by their own testimony."[78] For Calvin, the content of the natural law that conscience apprehends is basically the same as the content of the Ten Commandments,[79] and it is this apprehension that allows conscience to serve as "a certain mean between God and man, because it does not allow man to suppress within himself what he knows, but pursues him to the point of convicting him."[80]

Modern Christian theological discussions of conscience have been dominated by Roman Catholic voices, both because of differences in how conscience is conceptualized in Catholic and Protestant traditions and because of general theological differences in Catholic and Protestant ethics. A central difference arises from the way Catholic moral theology focuses attention on individual sins (and their particularized implications for the sacrament of penance), while Protestant thought is more concerned with an individual's sinfulness in general and its need for wholesale confession and forgiveness.[81] Such differences can be detected historically in the contrast between Luther and Calvin, who saw conscience as that which convicts a person of his sin before God, and Aquinas, who described conscience as a part of practical reason whose function is to facilitate moral decision making. These historical differences make it less surprising to encounter David Little's comment that one would labor in vain to find an extended discussion of conscience among major modern Protestant theologians (e.g., Karl Barth, Dietrich Bonhoeffer, Emil Brunner, and Reinhold Niebuhr).[82] Though extended treatments may not exist among such authors, it is interesting to note that when conscience is addressed by Barth, for instance, it is defined in terms of the encounter between God's command and human action in concrete circumstances and choices. For Barth, conscience pertains to our responsiveness (obedience) to God's command, rather than an independent human ability to apprehend and follow moral reasoning.[83] For Bonhoeffer, conscience signifies to humans that they are in disunion

78 Calvin, *Institutes of the Christian religion*, 282.

79 Ibid., 367–68.

80 Ibid., 848.

81 James M. Gustafson, *Protestant and Roman Catholic ethics: prospects for rapprochement* (Chicago: University of Chicago Press, 1978), 3.

82 Little, "A view of conscience within the Protestant theological tradition," 20–21.

83 Karl Barth, *Church dogmatics*, vol. III.4 (Edinburgh: T. & T. Clark, 1961), 8–9, 382.

with themselves,[84] and the awareness of this disunion results in autonomous (and therefore futile) efforts of "natural conscience" to reject evil and pursue good based on a knowledge of good and evil. In contrast to the futility of natural conscience, Bonhoeffer understood faith in Christ as creating a new kind of conscience that offers the only means for achieving true unity with oneself.[85] For Barth and Bonhoeffer, conscience is intimately related to the human need for God and requires a responsiveness to God through faith and obedience.

Roman Catholic views of conscience focus heavily on the cognitive dimension, whereby moral reasoning results in practical conclusions representing the application of basic moral principles to the real world.[86] Mention is sometimes made of another level of conscience in the Roman Catholic tradition that represents *being* more than *doing*, which may be referred to as "transcendental conscience." This represents an individual's deeply personal awareness of herself in relation to God that communicates to the individual what it means to be fully human.[87]

In Eastern Orthodox Christianity, there is an emphasis both on conscience as the consciousness of God and on its capacity to judge between good and evil.[88] Different strands of Eastern Orthodoxy offer various interpretations of the impact that sin has on that judging capacity. Some maintain that the innate ability of conscience to distinguish between good and evil has been obscured by human sin and requires divine revelation before conscience is able to do its intended work. Others, like Chrysostom, are more sanguine about the potential of innate conscience to make accurate moral judgments according to the dictates of natural law. These latter views resonate with Roman Catholic assessments by stressing that all human beings are endowed by God with a moral capacity that enables them to distinguish and choose between virtue and vice.[89]

In contrast to the New Testament, the Hebrew Bible does not have a word for conscience. Maurer attributes this fact to the Hebrew understanding of the immediacy of the relationship between God's Word – which is in the mouth and heart of God's people (Deuteronomy

[84] Dietrich Bonhoeffer, *Ethics* (New York: Macmillan, 1955), 24.
[85] Ibid., 243–44.
[86] William E. May, *An introduction to moral theology* (Huntington, IN: Our Sunday Visitor, Inc., 2003), 58–59.
[87] Ibid., 60.
[88] Stephen Thomas, "Conscience in Orthodox thought," in *Conscience in world religions*, ed. Jayne Hoose (Notre Dame, IN: University of Notre Dame Press, 1999), 106–17.
[89] Ibid., 117.

30:14) – and the human response to that Word.[90] Instead of conscience supplying some sort of rational interface between God's will and human obedience, there is an awareness of the need for direct responsiveness to God's will by adhering to His statutes. It should also be said that the Hebrew scriptures refer to the "heart" in a way that parallels the Christian idea of conscience, for the heart represents the inner self that contains a person's thoughts, judgments, and motivations and that, when enlightened by God, gains wisdom.[91]

Within the Jewish tradition there is ambivalence regarding the heart's potential to provide reliable moral guidance, since its promptings cannot always be trusted. This weakness is remedied by the revealed truth of Torah, the law, which serves as the trustworthy moral guide to distinguishing between good and evil. In the ultimate moral vision for the Jew, there is a union of these two parts, Torah and the heart, within the will of God.[92] Torah serves as the foundation for the legal tradition at the center of classical Judaism, in which rabbinical interpretation employs reason to expound on revealed truth and in which the discipline of law (*halakha*) cultivates an informed conscience that grows in independence even as it maintains its (potentially tense) relation to and respect for authority.[93] The rabbinical tradition entails a notable integration of authority, reason, and law, and the combination of these three features points to a parallel between traditional Judaism and Roman Catholic Christianity that does not apply to Protestant Christianity: in both Judaism and Catholicism, a person with authority (rabbi or priest) interprets a body of law (Torah or canon law) in order to make wise determinations (as a judge or confessor).[94]

Islam appears to take a dimmer view of the capacity of conscience apart from divine revelation, but conscience enlightened by divine revelation is able to discern the moral quality of our thoughts, words, and actions, and accompanies that discernment with pleasing or painful feelings depending on their good or bad quality.[95] But because human discernment on its own limited strength is incapable of nonarbitrary moral assessment,

90 Maurer, "† σύνοιδα, † συνείδησις," 908.

91 Grisez and Shaw, "Conscience: knowledge of moral truth," 41–42.

92 Jonathan Gorsky, "Conscience in Jewish tradition," in *Conscience in world religions*, ed. Hoose, 130–31.

93 Ibid., 138–39.

94 Gustafson, *Protestant and Roman Catholic ethics*, 2.

95 Ron Geaves, "Islam and conscience," in *Conscience in world religions*, ed. Hoose, 155–57.

divine law is needed to provide the standard against which human actions are judged. Accordingly, divine revelation must be brought to bear on every activity.[96]

The religious beliefs that have defined traditional understandings of conscience help explain how conscience and religious faith have become intertwined in modern society. This is particularly true in the United States, where religious liberty has historically been understood to involve sacred rights of conscience.[97] The interweaving of conscience and religious belief arises because conscience concerns fundamental human beliefs about truth, meaning, and purpose that determine actions by individuals and groups. In the United States, questions of conscience have routinely overlapped questions of religious belief and practice, because religion has been the traditional framework in which beliefs and commitments related to truth, meaning, and purpose have been communicated. Of course, this need not be so. Nonreligious beliefs of fundamental human significance have also served as grounds for claims of conscience. But history shows that while not dependent on a religious grounding, conscience has been so closely associated with religious concerns that, at least in the United States, a preferential treatment of specifically religious beliefs has developed in matters pertaining to conscience. This preferential treatment is illustrated by the observation that the framers of the U.S. Constitution chose to protect the free exercise of religion rather than the free exercise of conscience, making it clear that legal protection in the United States "would not extend to secular claims of conscience."[98]

V. RELATING CONSCIENCE TO PRACTICAL WISDOM THROUGH MORAL REASONING AND MOTIVATION

In historical and modern writings, it appears to be difficult to find clear descriptions or analyses of the relationship between conscience and practical wisdom. Nevertheless, their shared conceptual territory can be seen in the way they both involve moral beliefs and values, reason, deliberation regarding concrete circumstances, motivation to act on what one

[96] Ibid., 161.

[97] Daniel L. Dreisbach and Mark David Hall, eds., *The sacred rights of conscience: selected readings on religious liberty and church–state relations in the American founding* (Indianapolis: Liberty Fund, 2009).

[98] Michael W. McConnell, "The origins and historical understanding of free exercise of religion," *Harvard Law Review* 103, no. 7 (1990): 1410.

believes to be true, and the significance of moral agency and identity as expressed by notions of moral integrity (integrity will be discussed in Chapter 6).

One example of how conscience can be seen in relation to practical wisdom is found in Aquinas. As already noted, he viewed conscience not as a virtue (disposition), but as the application of knowledge to activity (applying general principles to individual cases). This is very similar to the way prudence functions in his philosophy. Langston notes direct links in Aquinas between these two entities, since prudence responds to the dictates of conscience, and conscience is informed by the secondary moral principles apprehended by prudence.[99] This suggests a mutual relationship that has a circularity about it. Another link between conscience and practical wisdom in Aquinas is a shared dependence on the ability to grasp certain self-evident truths (called *synderesis*) – whether the basic moral principles necessary for conscience or the ultimate human ends necessary for practical wisdom.[100] D'Arcy finds this dependence on *synderesis* problematic in Aquinas, because Aquinas failed to tell us which moral principles are shared by all human beings (i.e., which ones are part of the universal natural law). As a result, says D'Arcy, we are left wondering how extensive the common moral ground of conscience is presumed to be.[101] As a more general criticism, D'Arcy cites the work of Deman to suggest that Aquinas simply did not provide an adequate account of the relationship between conscience and practical wisdom.[102] But these controversies aside, a relationship between conscience and practical wisdom appears to be present in the Catholic tradition, as is suggested by the Catechism's portrayal of conscience as including *synderesis* and being closely associated with prudence, since it is prudence that "immediately guides the judgment of conscience" by directing the application of moral principles in individual cases.[103]

The challenge of identifying features that distinguish conscience from practical wisdom is perhaps what causes some writers to underplay or remove any differences. For instance, Grisez and Shaw believe that the function of a mature conscience is to answer the question "What is the good and wise thing to do?"[104] Similarly, Hardt claims that in Aquinas acts

99 Langston, *Conscience and other virtues*: 43.
100 D'Arcy, *Conscience and its right to freedom*, 70.
101 Ibid., 71.
102 Ibid., 135.
103 Langston, *Conscience and other virtues*, 110–11.
104 Grisez and Shaw, "Conscience: knowledge of moral truth," 41.

of conscience are "constituted by the making of reasonable decisions in light of moral norms, practical considerations, and contextual facts" and concludes that conscience is "the human mind making moral judgments about a practical course of action."[105] When conscience is thus described as reasoned decision making within a moral framework, it clearly resembles the virtue of practical wisdom. So perhaps it is not surprising to find that Pieper, speaking within the Thomistic tradition, concludes that the living unity of *synderesis* and prudence "is nothing less than the thing we commonly call 'conscience.'"[106]

An alternative assessment would incline in the opposite direction, denying any substantial overlap between conscience and practical wisdom and separating their activities, especially by emptying conscience of any deliberative function. Such a view can be seen in the way Fuss portrays conscience as *merely* a matter of integrating moral belief and action, rather than a much broader view that includes belief–action integration *and* moral reasoning. For Fuss, conscience is a matter of living with a driving sense of integrity that disposes us to act on our moral judgments, rather than the process of reaching those judgments through practical reasoning in the first place.[107] Between the alternatives of overlap and separation, Langston suggests that conscience should be seen as intimately and thoroughly related to the virtues, especially practical wisdom, and to their cultivation.[108] This is not surprising, given that Langston adopts Broad's understanding of conscience as having three dimensions – moral reasoning, moral emotion, and moral motivation – at least two of which (reasoning and motivation) are central to traditional concepts of practical wisdom.

VI. SUMMARY

The concept of conscience has a complex history extending over two thousand years. The Christian tradition incorporated the Greek idea that conscience is that universal human experience of inner pain related to actions that go against human nature, even as Christianity also recognized that conscience is limited by the fallibility and finiteness of human understanding. In the Catholic tradition, conscience is a form of practical

[105] Hardt, "The conscience debate," 153–54.
[106] Pieper, *The four cardinal virtues*, 11.
[107] Fuss, "Conscience," 47.
[108] Langston, *Conscience and other virtues*, 174–75.

reasoning about moral issues that consciously applies knowledge to action and can even be understood in a syllogistic fashion – we grasp self-evident, basic moral principles (major premise); we make judgments about an action within a given set of circumstances (minor premise); and we draw conclusions about the goodness or badness of that action (conclusion). As a matter of moral reasoning, conscience represents one's best moral judgment. This explains why its conclusions are seen as nonnegotiable, because one can do no better in the moral life than one's best – *even if* the conclusions of conscience in a given case happen to be, from some superior moral perspective, mistaken.

After the Reformation, Protestant understandings of conscience shifted the focus from the moral status of actions to the spiritual status of persons. On this view, the primary purpose of conscience was to allow an individual to see his entire self as standing before the judgment of God, either as guilty (because unrepentant) or as saved (because repentant and forgiven). Subsequent understandings of conscience included Joseph Butler's influential promotion of conscience as a moral faculty that perceives right and wrong immediately without requiring rational deliberation, thereby functioning like a private moral sense organ endowed by God to represent in humans God's infallible moral commands. A similarly instinct-like idea of conscience was suggested by Kant, who viewed it as a universal, internal moral judge. With the exception of the enduring Catholic view, by the nineteenth and twentieth centuries there emerged a view of conscience as a faculty, separated from practical reason and serving as an infallible, directing, and punitive guarantor of morality.

Contemporary assessments of conscience have been diverse, ranging from the traditional Catholic view to the widely affirmed three-dimensional interpretation of C. D. Broad, which involves moral cognition (reasoning), morally directed emotion, and moral motivation. A contrasting view holds that conscience does not fundamentally involve moral reasoning, but only moral motivation, such that the function of conscience is simply to motivate us to do what we believe is right and good; that is, it motivates us to make our actions consistent with our knowledge and beliefs, whatever they may be. Though notions of conscience that exclude moral reasoning and the capacity for critical reflection are questionable, the idea that conscience demands consistency between belief and action is an important insight.

There are considerable implications for medicine and ethics if we agree that conscience is intimately related to moral reasoning. A capacity that integrally involves reasoning cannot plausibly be categorized as merely a private moral sensibility; rather, it ought to be seen as something that can facilitate communication and understanding between persons and contribute to moral dialogue in professional and public spheres. Reason makes conscience accessible to other persons, open to interpersonal criticism, and open to the possibility of reason-compelling revision.

In traditions that view conscience as part of reason, attention is also given to the relationship between the conclusions of our deliberations and our motivation to act on those conclusions. The integration of reason and will in conscience resonates with the philosophical belief that when we take a moral claim to be true we also believe that it should be acted upon. By integrating reason and will, conscience encompasses a domain of belief – that is, moral conviction – that requires action, with the result that the motivation to act is inseparable from the ability to reach a conclusion. The relationship between reason and will in conscience parallels the relationship between deliberation and motivation in practical wisdom. Similarity between conscience and practical wisdom can also be found in the way they depend on a background of moral beliefs and values, engage concrete circumstances, and emphasize moral integration. In the Catholic tradition, there is so much similarity between conscience and practical wisdom (or prudence) that some commentators consider them nearly indistinguishable.

5

The Authority, Fallibility, and Normative Reach of Conscience

Conscience has been interpreted in a variety of ways throughout history, and some of these interpretations persist to the present day. In contemporary understandings, conscience tends to encompass three interwoven dimensions – moral cognition (reasoning), moral emotion, and moral motivation. Since these dimensions were discussed in the preceding chapter, we will now go on to consider other important features of conscience and their implications. These features include the authority and fallibility of conscience, the formation of conscience, the relationship between individual conscience and community, and the capacity of conscience to reach, as it were, from the individual to other persons by means of moral reasoning.

I. AUTHORITY OF CONSCIENCE

There is a paradox at the center of conscience that arises from its combination of two seemingly contradictory characteristics. On the one hand, conscience is understood to be uniquely authoritative, since it represents a person's most compelling and binding moral understanding; but on the other hand, it is admittedly fallible, since it is capable of directing a person to a conclusion or decision that she may subsequently acknowledge to have been morally bad or wrong.

Key to understanding the paradox of conscience is realizing that its vulnerability to error does not weaken its authority. The sovereign authority of an individual's conscience arises from the moral significance *for the individual* of conscience itself, *not* from the rational validity of its dictates as judged by other persons. Of course, it is hoped that a person acting conscientiously will make a sincere effort to inform his conscience by considering sources of moral understanding that both he and others understand to be valid. But the moral significance of conscience is fundamentally independent of other persons, because it relates directly to a person's moral freedom and dignity. The sovereign character of the *subjective authority* of conscience for the individual is especially evident in religious belief and practice. For example, Jacques Maritain insists that the human person is "free to choose his religious path at his own risk," for "his freedom of conscience is a natural, inviolable right."[1] The protection of this freedom is built into the foundation of liberal democracies as a sacred right.[2] And what is true for conscience regarding religious belief and practice is also true for morality, whether framed in religious or philosophical terms, for the authority of conscience creates a sense of moral necessity that compels a person to do what she believes is right, even if doing so incurs opposition.

Familiarity with rights of conscience in liberal democracies may make it easy to accept that conscience should be surrounded by protections that guard individuals against coercion from external powers. But the acceptability of such protective boundaries for conscience should not be allowed to create the false impression that by respecting rights of conscience we are treating its dictates as if they themselves were somehow self-justifying due to their origins. If the dictates of conscience were self-justifying, this would imply that conscience is entitled to disregard potential sources of moral truth that are external to the individual, whether communicated by other persons, societies, or traditions.

Martin Luther was aware of the risk of attributing self-justification to conscience – notwithstanding that his own life was a paradigmatic expression of the exercise of conscience in the face of threatening opposition from political and ecclesiastical powers. Luther believed that all persons are endowed by God with an understanding of the natural law that allows conscience to comprehend an objective source of moral truth. But Luther also believed that evil in the human heart and mind can so obscure the natural law that some persons are no longer able to follow it and are therefore deprived of an objective moral guide for action. He also believed that false teaching may lead to the formation of a mistaken conscience. For Luther, these liabilities of conscience had one remedy – the Word of God as revealed in the Bible. Without this external standard, he believed that conscience

[1] Jacques Maritain, *The rights of man and natural law* (New York: Gordian Press, 1971), 82.
[2] Dreisbach and Hall, *The sacred rights of conscience.*

would lack a solid ground for justification and could be misled by a person's own feelings.[3]

In contrast to Luther, Butler's religious anthropology delivered a far more optimistic conception of conscience, ascribing to it "that candle of the Lord within" that provides the capacity not only for moral reason but also for divine reason.[4] For Butler, the dictates of conscience have compelling authority because conscience is a capacity that comes with its own guarantee.[5] The self-justifying nature of conscience is a recurring theme in the Christian theological tradition because of a belief that, in some vital way, conscience represents the voice or light of God in human beings. Seen this way, conscience is "a sacred, sovereign authority that must be engaged, consulted, and obeyed as one would obey God."[6] Joseph Ratzinger (Pope Emeritus Benedict XVI) gestures toward this view when maintaining that conscience expresses "the thought of a kind of co-knowledge of man with God, and precisely from here there emerges the absoluteness with which conscience asserts its superiority over any and all authorities."[7] However, he joins with Spaemann in cautioning against any tendency to equate "individual judgments of conscience with the voice of God,"[8] and he holds that conscience is misunderstood if it is used to reduce morality to a merely subjective dimension and allowed to assume a completely independent, self-justifying character. While conscience is a crucial source of moral knowledge for Ratzinger, he objects to attempts to employ it as "a sort of deification of subjectivity, a rock of bronze on which even the magisterium is shattered."[9]

The problem of subjectivity regarding the authority of conscience can also be described in terms of moral individualism. Some who oppose giving conscience too much privilege may fear that too much respect for conscientious practice may facilitate a moral individualism that disregards social responsibilities and may justify positions that are the result of idiosyncratic personal preferences rather than valid moral commitments. This is a serious concern, especially if conscience is conceived as a private moral monitor rather than a form of moral reasoning. It is a concern reflected in the analysis of moral individualism by Charles Taylor

[3] Zachman, *The assurance of faith*, 26–28.
[4] Hebblethwaite, *Ethics and religion in a pluralistic age*, 44.
[5] Ibid., 47–48.
[6] Callahan, *In good conscience*, 34.
[7] Ratzinger, *On conscience*, 51–52.
[8] Ibid., 60.
[9] Ibid., 51.

in *The Ethics of Authenticity*. Individualism, says Taylor, has given rise to a morally prescriptive form of relativism grounded in a principle of mutual self-respect, according to which "everyone has a right to develop their own form of life, grounded on their own sense of what is really important or of value."[10] He calls this the individualism of self-fulfillment and sees in it a debased but still potent version of the moral ideal of being true to oneself, of being an authentic self. The desire for authenticity in the moral life derives from a sense that morality has an internal voice within each of us that anchors our moral understanding. Though Taylor believes that the search for authenticity is valid, the problem with its debased form – the individualism of self-fulfillment – is that the "moral accent" of authenticity has been displaced. Originally, the inner moral voice was believed to be important because it allowed us to be in touch with our moral feelings about an external source (e.g., God or the idea of the good) and thereby guided us to act rightly.[11] However, the subjectivist turn in modern culture has made connection with something deep within us a purpose unto itself, making authenticity a matter of finding out what being human means "for me."[12]

Taylor argues that the individualism of self-fulfillment is self-defeating because it disregards the demands of our ties to others and because it disregards demands from anything or anyone beyond our own human desires or aspirations. He believes that such disregard destroys the conditions necessary for realizing genuine authenticity, because authenticity requires a horizon of significance beyond oneself that makes an individual's choices meaningful. Based on his interpretation of what constitutes moral significance, his analysis opposes those who suggest that because an option is freely chosen, choice itself confers worth.[13] The ideal of self-choice makes sense only because some options and issues are more significant than others. To disregard demands beyond the self is to trivialize moral decision making and to suppress the very conditions of moral significance. Taylor concludes his argument by describing the connection between authenticity and personal identity, which is based on the moral background that sustains them both. "Only if I exist in a world in which history, or the demands of nature, or the needs of my fellow human beings, or the duties of citizenship, or the call of God, or something else

[10] Charles Taylor, *The ethics of authenticity* (Cambridge, MA: Harvard University Press, 1991), 14.
[11] Ibid., 26.
[12] Ibid., 29.
[13] Ibid., 38.

of this order *matters* crucially, can I define an identity for myself that is not trivial."[14]

Taylor's analysis of moral individualism reminds us that there are weighty reasons to believe that reference to conscience by itself should never be taken to be an automatic, self-justifying moral maneuver, no matter how much sincerity or authenticity may be claimed for conscience. Instead, we should expect persons who make conscience-based claims to describe how their moral beliefs and commitments are related to their moral positions and choices – which is to say that we should expect some degree of explanation or reasoning when claims of conscience are introduced to discussions about ethical decision making.

Despite concerns about the potential for inordinate subjectivity, the dictates of conscience are nevertheless appropriately understood to be genuinely authoritative for the person whose conscience is at issue. One way to defend this authority is to identify conscience with moral belief and action and argue that if conscience represents the process whereby an individual acts on the moral beliefs he accepts as true, then conscience simply has to be authoritative.[15] For if it is agreed that conscience depends fundamentally on moral beliefs and if it is agreed that inherent in accepting a moral belief as true is accepting the need to act on that belief, then conscience can be seen as that which authorizes and compels actions that express the moral beliefs one takes to be true. Seen this way, conscience produces an imperative that is at the heart of moral agency and provides an immediate cause for moral action. It is an unavoidable imperative, since conscience must have the last word as the ultimate *subjective* norm of morality for an individual,[16] given the responsibility an individual has to act according to the moral beliefs and assessments she takes to be true.

The subjective authority of conscience invites us to question how an individual's conscience and its judgments are formed and on what grounds the guiding beliefs of conscience are taken to be true. These considerations raise questions of epistemology – that is, how it is that we are justified in taking beliefs to be true – and bear directly on the relationship between the subjective and objective dimensions of a person's conscience and the extent to which the authority of conscience should be respected when its exercise affects other people.

[14] Ibid., 40–41.
[15] Duncan-Jones, "The notion of conscience," 126.
[16] Dolan, "Conscience in the Catholic theological tradition," 12.

The case of Martin Luther, albeit unique in its historical significance and drama, illustrates what is at stake in the interplay between the subjective and objective dimensions of conscience. Driven by conscience to stand his theological ground, he found himself on trial for heresy before the highest sacred and secular powers of his day, including Charles, the Holy Roman Emperor. Luther's interrogator asked, "Do you or do you not repudiate your books and the errors they contain?" Luther's response reveals the core substance of his belief about conscience:

> "Since then Your Majesty and your lordships desire a simple reply, I will answer without horns and without teeth. Unless I am convicted by Scripture and plain reason – I do not accept the authority of popes and councils, for they have contradicted each other – my conscience is captive to the Word of God. I cannot and I will not recant anything, for to go against conscience is neither right nor safe. God help me. Amen." The earliest printed version [of this event] added the words: "Here I stand, I cannot do otherwise."[17]

Luther did not treat conscience as self-justifying. Instead, he indicated that the moral validity of conscience rested on external sources – either the revealed truth of scripture or the capacity of human reason.

Reliance on reason to apprehend moral truth fits well with contemporary practices of moral justification, but the suggestion that conscience could rely on an external source such as the Bible might be seen by some as a capitulation to external authority or tradition that would compromise one's moral autonomy. Such a compromise might seem to undermine the authenticity of conscience itself, if it is taken to represent unthinking obedience rather than conscientious freedom. However, an alternative view would suggest that a morally serious person can accept the authority of an external source without diminishing his own autonomy, so long as the validity of that source's authority has been justified in his mind. As Langston observes, personal autonomy is not compromised if an external authority is accepted autonomously.[18]

II. FALLIBILITY OF CONSCIENCE

Claims about the authority of conscience can also be criticized on the basis of its fallibility. How can conscience be authoritative in a morally valid sense when it is susceptible to errors of fact, reasoning, and moral

[17] Roland H. Bainton, *Here I stand: a life of Martin Luther* (New York: Mentor Books, 1950), 144.

[18] Langston, *Conscience and other virtues*, 130.

perspective? This is an urgent question in light of the capacity humans have for self-deception, a capacity so large that war criminals like Himmler[19] and Eichmann[20] perpetrated horrific evils with a self-reported "clear" conscience, and even out of a self-perceived sense of duty. The fallibility of conscience runs like a fault line through its proposed authority, and it can be criticized on religious grounds because it puts "something human and fallible in the place of the divine law" or on nonreligious grounds because it risks "exalting prejudice or some ideologically blinkered judgement or reaction."[21] Such criticisms underscore how unsettling the combination of authority and fallibility in conscience can appear, and it calls for clarification.

It is generally accepted that conscience can err, in that the actions it authorizes are not necessarily good or right in a nonsubjective sense. This is readily confirmed by the heinous acts perpetrated "conscientiously" by persons such as Himmler and Eichmann, or by the observation that some individuals report that certain actions they have carried out in good conscience turn out, in retrospect and by their own admission, to have been bad or wrong.

If conscience is conceived primarily as a part of practical moral reasoning, its capacity for error can arise directly from the potential for mistakes in perception or reasoning. One can misunderstand pertinent facts, draw mistaken conclusions based on those misunderstood facts, or misinterpret or misapply moral virtues or principles that are relevant.[22] Conscience can also fail to grasp the wider moral framework relevant to a situation, especially when that framework is part of a moral tradition.[23] But conscience can also be misled by self-deception and rationalization, a point that led Bonhoeffer to conclude that a person "whose only support is his conscience can never understand that a bad conscience may be healthier and stronger than a conscience which is deceived."[24] Such deception may arise when a person uses conscience as a subjective shell of protection against criticism and acts as if sincerity signifies the presence of a morally correct conscience – especially when it is accompanied by the subjective experience of peace and joy[25] or the absence of doubts or

[19] D'Arcy, "Conscience."
[20] Fuss, "Conscience," 48–50.
[21] Hebblethwaite, *Ethics and religion in a pluralistic age*, 37.
[22] Pellegrino, "The physician's conscience, conscience clauses, and religious belief," 227.
[23] Pierce, *Conscience in the New Testament*, 88–89.
[24] Bonhoeffer, *Ethics*, 66.
[25] Curran, "Conscience in the light of the Catholic moral tradition," 18.

scruples.[26] Deception of this kind entails the false assumption that remorse or contentment is the guarantor of moral impropriety or rectitude, respectively. Conscience will always be vulnerable to mistakes in moral reasoning, weaknesses in moral character, and the possibility of self-deception. This explains why conscience should never be treated as if it were beyond the boundaries of questioning, explaining, and dialogue.[27]

As an illustration of the concern about self-deception, consider the problem of conflicts of interest in health care. Conflicts of interest are a particularly salient context in which some physicians may be at risk of self-deception, as manifested through rationalization or denial. The authors of one study found that some physicians lack the ability to resolve the cognitive dissonance they manifest when defending their interactions with pharmaceutical representatives, while simultaneously recognizing the inherent conflicts of interest these interactions pose.[28] The possibility of self-deception among physicians indicates the importance of the responsibility the medical profession and society have to ensure – through guidelines, policies, and regulations – that physicians avoid practices that undermine their fiduciary obligations to patients, such as when a secondary financial interest exerts undue influence on the primary interest of patient welfare.[29]

The conclusions of conscience have generally been understood to be binding for the individual, even though it is recognized that conscience is a potentially flawed source of moral guidance because of its vulnerability to error. Among some proponents, this understanding is so strong that it results in an absolute imperative: one should always, without exception, follow conscience. How this imperative can withstand the paradox of conscience – that something intrinsically fallible can be inherently authoritative – becomes apparent when the cognitive dimension of conscience is understood to be a matter of moral reasoning. The implications of the rational dimension of conscience are clarified in the writing of Aquinas, for instance, when he describes the authority of conscience as arising from the twofold belief that conscience is a manifestation of reason, and reason is always to be followed, whether reason is, in actual

[26] Ratzinger, *On conscience*, 16–17.

[27] William C. Spohn, "Conscience and moral development," in *Conscience*, ed. Curran, 133.

[28] S. C. Chimonas, T. A. Brennan, and D. J. Rothman, "Physicians and drug representatives: exploring the dynamics of the relationship," *Journal of General Internal Medicine* 22 (2007): 184–90.

[29] Institute of Medicine, *Conflict of interest in medical research, education, and practice*, 46.

fact, right or wrong.[30] For Aquinas, reason is always to be followed because it "presents its judgment as true and as issuing from God, the author of all truth."[31] Of course, one need not invoke religious justifications in order to take reason seriously. Frankena, for example, speaks in philosophical terms by recognizing the conclusions of conscience as binding because they are the final and best assessment of what a person believes is right, even if that assessment might in fact be wrong. For Frankena, conscience is not self-justifying, but it is still true that conscience must be followed:

> [A] man must in the moment of decision do what he thinks is right. He cannot do otherwise. This does not mean that what he does will be right or even that he will not be worthy of blame or punishment. He simply has no choice, for he cannot at that moment see any discrepancy between what is right and what he thinks is right.[32]

The sense of having no choice but to do as conscience dictates is also emphasized by Grisez and Shaw, who point out that if a person's conscience is mistaken, he is simply not in a position to know it.[33] There is a certain tautological quality to conscience in this regard, for conscience in the traditions represented by these writers is understood to be that which crystallizes and completes the process of moral deliberation as it leads to moral action. It is by definition the culmination of a person's best effort to understand what is morally good and right in the circumstances at hand. As May puts it, a "person has the obligation to follow his or her conscience – i.e., to act in accordance with his or her own best judgment of what he or she is to do – precisely because this judgment of conscience is the final judgment that a person makes about the moral goodness or badness of the alternatives possible for him or her."[34]

If it is agreed that a person is always obligated to follow her conscience, it might seem that a person should not be held morally responsible for conscientious choices that lead to wrong actions. This raises an old question about the exculpatory nature of conscience, which led Kant to the following conclusion: "If a man's conscience errs and he acts in accordance with it, his acts may be at fault, but they cannot be accounted to him

30 Davies, *The thought of Thomas Aquinas*, 236.
31 Aquinas, *Summa theologica*, 197.
32 Frankena, *Ethics*, 60.
33 Grisez and Shaw, "Conscience: knowledge of moral truth," 43.
34 May, *An introduction to moral theology*, 61.

for a transgression."[35] The Catholic tradition addresses this issue by considering the extent to which conscience has been properly informed and whether any misinformation that has led to moral error was due to voluntary or involuntary ignorance. The distinction between voluntary and involuntary ignorance arises from the belief that each person has a responsibility to ensure that his or her conscience is properly informed so that preventable errors in moral reasoning are not committed out of negligence. Wrong actions committed without negligence are therefore excusable. As Aquinas remarks, "mistakes that arise without negligence from ignorance of some circumstance can make resulting acts of will involuntary and thus excuse them."[36] On this account, a person is morally responsible (and should feel remorse) for a conscientiously motivated wrong action if he has willfully neglected the responsibility to pursue, consider, and incorporate empirical facts, moral values, or sources of guidance that could and should have been known to be relevant. However, if a person has not willfully neglected this responsibility, but nevertheless comes to realize that he has acted with an involuntarily misinformed conscience, he will have cause for regret (but not remorse), as well as grounds for addressing whatever deficiencies of knowledge or understanding led to the involuntary mistake.[37] The distinction between voluntary and involuntary mistakes in conscience within the Catholic tradition, associated with the contrasting experiences of remorse and regret, can be seen as paralleling the distinction between culpability and responsibility in the moral life.

By now it should be very evident how important it is to distinguish between the individual authority of conscience and its fallibility. The authority of conscience arises from its intimate relationship with moral freedom and human dignity, which explains why individual conscience has been held in such high regard by societies that have come to respect it as an inviolable human attribute. But alongside this authority is fallibility, a weakness that arises from the ramifications of human finitude (failures in apprehension and understanding) and the powers of self-deception. It is this intrinsic fallibility that cautions against suggestions that conscience is somehow self-justifying with respect to truth. As Granrose observes, relatively few people have ever claimed that conscience was in fact infallible, and far more have claimed that conscience has an authority that justifies the conclusion that its unique demands on the individual should

35 Kant, *Lectures on ethics*, 132.

36 Aquinas, *Summa theologica*, 197.

37 May, *An introduction to moral theology*, 63.

override other competing moral concerns.[38] The importance of being clear on the distinction between the authority and fallibility of conscience is at times brought to light by its neglect. For instance, when critics of conscientious practice in health care criticize some advocates of the freedom of conscience for interpreting conscience as "the guide to universal truth,"[39] they would help their readers by acknowledging the distinction between authority and fallibility. Doing so would expand the grounds of debate to include the recognition that the fallibility of conscience is traditionally understood to coexist with an enormously high degree of respect for its authority, regardless of the actual rightness or wrongness of the actions it motivates.

III. FORMATION OF CONSCIENCE

If conscience is to function properly, it has to be properly informed so as to minimize its susceptibility to error. The need to be informed implies that a conscientious action comes with a moral responsibility to pursue, consider, and incorporate empirical facts and moral values that are known to be relevant or to seek advice from reliable sources of moral guidance when the need for such assistance is recognized. But in addition to the moral responsibility to *inform* one's conscience when one is deliberating over details in specific situations, there is also a need to *form* one's conscience in general so that it is habitually less likely to succumb to error.

What does it mean to *form* one's conscience? In the Catholic tradition, the proper formation of conscience is accomplished through education within a moral or spiritual community and by reflection on sources of moral truth that are external to the individual. Within this tradition, the process of formation is understood to be an obligation, which, if neglected, can lead to harm because of the potential development of a conscience that has effectively become stunted, stamped out, and falsified.[40] Those who see conscience as a moral capacity that requires formation believe that individuals have a responsibility to cultivate their moral understanding – by reflecting on the formal teachings of their moral or spiritual community,[41] being open to the revealed Word of

38 John T. Granrose, "The authority of conscience," in *Conscience*, ed. Donnelly and Lyons, 223.

39 R. A. Charo, "The celestial fire of conscience: refusing to deliver medical care," *New England Journal of Medicine* 352 (2005): 2471–73.

40 Ratzinger, *On conscience*, 62.

41 Pellegrino, "The physician's conscience, conscience clauses, and religious belief."

God (for those who believe in the truth of sacred scriptures),[42] and being willing to learn from the moral values and exemplars of their own community and other morally serious and well-intentioned people.[43] The fulfillment of this responsibility of formation requires a desire to live a good life and make decisions that are motivated by one's best understanding of what moral goodness entails. This requires that conscience be teachable, since its formation depends on an internal motivation to enliven moral education through emotional attachment to moral exemplars and responsive engagement with moral narratives – all of which should encourage the integration of moral reasoning, moral emotions, and moral action.[44]

The need to form conscience by engaging moral narratives points to the relationship between moral formation and the humanities, especially literature. Sidney Callahan argues that the humanities are a vital moral resource, providing what she calls a "conscience curriculum" in which students learn vicariously from the moral decision making of other people, both fictional and real.[45] She draws a connection between the potential of the humanities to nurture conscience and the role of narrative in human understanding and communication, a connection that is particularly germane to medicine given the central and enduring place of case presentations (patient stories) in medical education and practice. Narratives help us attend to the complexity of individual lives in linear time so that we see more clearly how motivations, actions, and consequences are interwoven. By listening to moral narratives, we learn more about the significance of human intention and moral choice when individuals have to navigate the demands of time, persons, and place within the constraints of concrete circumstances. Callahan maintains that such listening instructs both the mind and the heart, as the moral imagination learns to consider the values at stake in a moment of decision. And empathic engagement with moral narratives helps form the thoughts and feelings of the listener that prepare her to respond conscientiously when required to make moral choices in the future.[46] When we consider the role moral narratives can play in the formation of conscience, we are reminded that they have been used for thousands of years, as evidenced by the Greek, medieval, and Renaissance cultivation of moral education

42 Curran, "Conscience in the light of the Catholic moral tradition," 21.
43 Ibid., 22.
44 Callahan, *In good conscience*, 208.
45 Ibid., 205–206.
46 Ibid., 207.

and character development through stories communicating moral images and exemplars to awaken in the listener a love for what is good.[47] The centrality of moral narrative to human experience and growth is summarized by MacIntyre's observation that human beings are – in their actions, practices, and fictions – essentially storytelling animals, such that if children are deprived of stories they become "unscripted, anxious stutterers in their actions and their words."[48]

In addition to the need for teachability, internal motivation, and engagement with moral narratives, commentators on conscience also see the need for *humility* in response to the problem of fallibility. Indeed, humility can be seen as perhaps the most fitting response to the paradoxical relationship between authority and fallibility in the function of conscience. Humility can facilitate a self-scrutinizing attitude that tempers the exercise of conscience and cultivates confidence without arrogance. If accompanied by humility, such confidence can be compatible with a readiness to learn from the experience of others, acknowledge prejudices, and modify judgments in light of more information or better insights.[49] Humility is encouraged by the awareness that one's conscience is in need of an external, objective norm of morality. In theistic moral traditions, the appreciation of this need entails a desire to bring conscience into conformity with the moral order created by God. This can be expressed as the desire to "do everything in our power to see to it that our judgments of conscience are informed and in accord with the moral order of which God is creator"[50] or as the desire to restore "the erring heart to its primeval affinity with the ideals of righteousness, justice, compassion and truth" and rekindle the holiness of God within human beings.[51]

The connection between understanding, reasoning, and motivation in the formation of conscience reminds us how closely conscience is related to the virtues – a closeness that is especially apparent when conscience is described in terms that resemble practical wisdom. Grisez and Shaw, for example, maintain that the formation of conscience requires three things: clarification of the moral principles known by natural law, awareness of realistic alternatives in a given situation, and an appreciation for the way in which moral principles are relevant to action.[52] This

47 Meilaender, *The theory and practice of virtue*, 54–55.
48 MacIntyre, *After virtue*, 216.
49 May, *An introduction to moral theology*, 63.
50 Ibid.
51 Gorsky, "Conscience in Jewish tradition," 150.
52 Grisez and Shaw, "Conscience: knowledge of moral truth," 46.

understanding of the formation of conscience not only incorporates the cognitive features of practical reason, but also encompasses the conative (motivational) features that characterize individuals who desire to live a conscientious life – individuals who increasingly want to do what is truly right and, in doing it, are able to integrate their selves around their choices and actions.[53]

IV. CONSCIENCE AND ITS RELATIONSHIP TO COMMUNITY

In Chapter 2, it was noted that moral community plays an essential role in educating individuals in virtue. This role is as vital in the formation of conscience as it is in the development of virtue, which is not surprising given the interrelationships between the two.

Stanley Hauerwas has been one of the more audible critics of approaches to moral reasoning that fail to acknowledge that the beliefs and practices of a person's moral community predetermine the way moral questions are understood and decided. He emphasizes the need to consider how moral problems are described and what paradigmatic moral examples are chosen to facilitate moral comparisons. He maintains that these descriptions and choices reflect the virtues and commitments of the moral and religious communities in which individuals live, think, and reason. There cannot be, he argues, any tradition-free account of practical reason or practical wisdom, because each moral community determines the way moral reflection occurs and is made intelligible. Moral questions cannot simply be answered by deducing conclusions from a set of free-standing moral principles, for it takes a moral community to interpret those principles in terms of the goods and goals they value.[54] Charles Taylor would agree, as is clear from his observation that all moral reasoning occurs within a community that determines such fundamental beliefs as who counts as a moral agent and is thereby worthy of respect and rights.[55]

The claim that writers like Hauerwas and Taylor make – that moral reflection and understanding depend on moral community – is equally relevant to the formation and function of conscience. Sometimes this aspect of conscience is noted when attention is called to its social

53 Ibid., 47.

54 Hauerwas, "Reconciling the practice of reason," 138–39.

55 Charles Taylor, "The diversity of goods," in *Utilitarianism and beyond*, ed. Amartya Sen and Bernard Williams (Cambridge: Cambridge University Press, 1982), 130–31.

dimension, on the grounds that we gain our moral bearings from our families, peers, adults, and religious and professional communities, carrying "their voices in our heads, for better or worse."[56] Communities create the web of social relationships in which individuals live, and this web influences the decisions of conscience. The community influence on the formation of conscience can also be understood as a feature of moral identity, which points to the socially embedded character of moral agency that is prominent in MacIntyre's analysis of the dependence of individuals on their moral traditions and cultures. On this analysis, an individual finds his moral identity in and through his membership in communities,[57] and this identity causes him to be accountable to particular people in that community, participate in critical moral deliberation, and acknowledge the individuality of other persons, all of which characterize moral agency.[58]

Langston describes the moral community's impact on the individual as a process whereby socially sanctioned norms are internalized within an individual's conscience, creating an equilibrium between the moral values of the community and the moral values of the individual. This process provides checks on individuals which ensure that they do not generally go against society's demands and that they do not slip into moral self-delusion.[59] And the two-way dynamic of this moral equilibrium means that individuals also influence their moral communities. As the norms of society influence the development of an individual's conscience, so also the words and actions of individuals sustain, challenge, or weaken the ethos of their community. Sidney Callahan underscores this point by noting that with "large and small moral decisions of conscience, we strengthen, or alternately erode and destroy, moral consciousness – in ourselves, in our families, and in our fellow sojourners."[60] When viewed in relation to moral communities and society, the highly individual aspect of conscience and its subjective authority are placed in context. Instead of independence and competition, one can acknowledge grounds for a dynamic interdependence between individual conscience and moral community. It is within this mutual relation that community provides individual conscience the moral resources necessary for its formation

56 Spohn, "Conscience and moral development," 133.
57 MacIntyre, *After virtue*, 84.
58 Alasdair MacIntyre, "Social structures and their threats to moral agency," *Philosophy* 74 (1995): 317.
59 Langston, *Conscience and other virtues*, 177.
60 Callahan, *In good conscience*, 214.

and function, and individual conscience contributes to the sustenance of moral community.

V. NORMATIVE REACH OF CONSCIENCE

To view the formation of conscience as a dynamic interplay between individuals and their moral communities is to invite consideration of how far beyond the individual the normative influence of her conscience should be expected or allowed to reach. Put another way, we can ask whether we should consider the conclusions of one person's conscience morally relevant to people other than herself.

To begin, we can consider this question in light of the discussion of the formation of conscience, which included the observation that one of the ways conscience is formed is through social interactions that help an individual see himself in relation to other selves and learn to appreciate the perspectives of other selves. This perspectival versatility can be summarily articulated by the golden rule – treating others as you would like them to treat you. Curran believes that the moral imperative expressed by the golden rule speaks directly to the formation of conscience, for it emphasizes the need to put oneself in another's position and see the situation from that person's perspective.[61] By shifting my perspective to that of another person, I avoid the tendency to place myself at the center of my own moral universe. The result of this perspectival shift can be seen as similar to what is achieved by the Kantian principle of universalizability, whereby there is a formal effort to detach moral judgments from tendencies toward partiality (especially partiality toward oneself). Langston makes substantially the same point by drawing from Kohlberg's belief that reversibility – the ability to see oneself in the position of others – is crucial in moral development.[62] In doing so he underscores a significant implication for conscience when it is capable of perspectival reversal: by allowing an individual to be sensitive to the perspectives and viewpoints of others, conscience does not merely function as a private moral monitor. Rather, it has a moral significance that extends beyond the individual because the dictates of one's conscience represent the dictates one would want all persons to follow.[63]

[61] Curran, "Conscience in the light of the Catholic moral tradition," 21.
[62] Langston, *Conscience and other virtues*, 175.
[63] Ibid., 175–76.

Another way in which to consider the question of normative reach refers us again to the status (subjective or objective) of truth as apprehended by the cognitive dimension of conscience through the capacity of moral reasoning. If the conclusions of a person's conscience are based on that person's subjective assessments, the moral relevance of those conclusions could legitimately be seen as limited to that person alone. Alternatively, if the conclusions of a person's conscience are based on objective moral claims, the moral relevance of those conclusions could legitimately be seen as applicable not only to that person but to other persons as well. Grisez, Shaw, and Ratzinger take the latter approach and situate conscience in direct relation to claims of truth and objectivity. On their accounts, conscience is informed by a moral reality that is external to the self and therefore has moral relevance beyond the boundaries of the self.

The subjective or objective relevance of conscience can also be considered in relation to the extent of its authority, as opposed to its apprehension of truth. Langston addresses this in his critique of Ryle's view of conscience as a person-specific, private monitor. He faults Ryle for "equating moral convictions with inclinations to behavior" and for failing to demonstrate that conscience has merely personal authority.[64] Langston grants that there is a unique link between a person and her own conscience (as opposed to others' consciences), but he attributes this uniqueness not to the relationship between a given person's conscience and the moral claims that flow from it, but to the relationship between a given person's conscience and that person's ability to control her own behavior in a way that she cannot (and should not) control the behavior of others. In short, Langston distinguishes between the authority of conscience and the authority of the *content* of conscience: "Although one's own conscience has a unique personal authority over one's own actions, the content of one's conscience has authority beyond the personal and extends to the behavior of others."[65]

In drawing this distinction, Langston calls our attention to the possibility that conscience can express a moral point of view that is generalizable to others if it is based on moral reasons that are reasonably perceived as equally relevant to all persons. For people who hold that conscience includes moral reasoning, it is entirely understandable that the conclusions of conscience should be portrayed as having more than merely

[64] Ibid., 97–98.
[65] Ibid., 98.

personal authority. In this regard, it is notable by way of contrast that Childress believes that people tend to invoke conscience not merely as a way to express moral reasoning, but as a personal motive-statement ("subjective rightness") *after* moral reasoning has failed to convince others of the "objective rightness" of a given course of action. This explains his conclusion that appeals to conscience tend to be a moral last resort.[66]

The relationship between conscience and the potential universalizability of its reasons and conclusions becomes particularly clear when conscience is guided by reasons that are expressed as moral principles. As Blustein notes, articulating the dictates of conscience in the language of moral reasoning and principles reminds us that just because an individual relies on conscience, it does not follow that the individual "must refrain from universalizing the moral standards that are determinative for his or her conscience."[67] Though conscience has direct implications for one's own actions in a way that it does not have for the actions of others – I am, but others are not, obligated to follow the dictates of *my* conscience – Blustein rightly observes that one person's conscience, if it entails moral reasoning, has universalizable implications. This is so because the universalizability of moral judgments is simply a standard feature of ethics, according to which "a person who believes that it is morally wrong for him or her to do something is also committed to judging that it is morally wrong for anyone in exactly similar or relevantly similar circumstances to do likewise."[68] This universalizability illuminates a similarity between conscience and what is referred to as the *moral point of view* – that impartial perspective of moral reasoning that considers oneself and one's interests to be morally equal (in relevant respects) to all other persons and their interests. Like the moral point of view, conscience can be seen as connecting an individual to the persons who surround that individual. To the extent that conscience articulates moral reasons that are impartial and universalizable, conscience has implications that extend beyond the individual, even if its dictates are, in fact, persuasive and authoritative only for the individual.

While the activity of conscience is frequently viewed in relation to beliefs, values, and reasons pertaining to the practical demands of moral decision making, there is a further aspect of conscience and its reach that pertains

66 Childress, "Appeals to conscience."

67 Jeffrey Blustein, "Doing what the patient orders: maintaining integrity in the doctor–patient relationship," *Bioethics* 7, no. 4 (1993): 289–314.

68 Ibid.

to the pursuit of our ultimate goals as human beings. This deeper aspect of conscience is evident in contemporary writers in political philosophy who view conscience as a fundamental expression of the human search for ultimate meaning and freedom. Nussbaum writes extensively about conscience in this respect, drawing heavily on Roger Williams's idea of conscience as a "faculty" in every person that "reasons, searches, and experiences emotions of longing" as it pursues questions of ultimate meaning.[69] Nussbaum suggests that regardless of our beliefs about religion, "we tend to believe that all human beings have moral and spiritual faculties and that these faculties, whether we call them 'conscience' or 'soul' or 'human dignity,' deserve respect wherever they are found" and, moreover, that these beliefs form "the basis of the modern human rights movement."[70] From our respect for conscience flows the conclusion that "we ought to respect the space required by any activity that has the general shape of searching for the ultimate meaning of life," limited only by the infringement of others' rights or compelling state interests.[71] For Nussbaum, conscience is an "infinitely precious" human characteristic that grounds human equality, demands universal respect, and justifies the argument for religious liberty and equality.[72] One sees a similarly high regard expressed in Rawls's theory of justice, in which parties in the "original position" are bound to agree on the equal liberty of conscience in light of the absolutely binding way that individuals who recognize religious and moral obligations experience the claims of those obligations on their actions.[73] In short, says Rawls, "[t]he question of equal liberty of conscience is settled. It is one of the fixed points of our considered judgments of justice."[74]

The normative reach of conscience is nicely illustrated by examples of its public expressions. Sidney Callahan observes that great moral heroes like Gandhi and Martin Luther King did not limit the dictates of their consciences to their own actions. On the contrary, they were compelled by conscience to intervene in the lives of others and the political process in general. Consistent with this observation, Callahan warns against the error of separating conscience from other kinds of moral decision

[69] Martha C. Nussbaum, *Liberty of conscience: in defense of America's tradition of religious equality* (New York: Basic Books, 2008), 168–69.
[70] Ibid., 52–53.
[71] Ibid., 169.
[72] Ibid., 19–20, 52–53.
[73] John Rawls, *A theory of justice* (Cambridge, MA: Harvard University Press, 1971), 205–208.
[74] Ibid., 206.

making, because to do so would mistakenly imply "that in narrow, very private domains, self-committed conscience can be active, but in interpersonal, social, and other moral questions, the same conscience must somehow disconnect from moral self-commitment and always be confined to operating in some self-absent, value-free mode."[75] This view is in accord with accounts of conscience that place reason in the foreground of its functioning, such as Langston's view that the moral reasoning of conscience implies that its moral authority is not merely personal but also applies, through the influence of moral argument, to the moral considerations of other persons.[76] Langston suggests not only that the conclusions of one's conscience should reflect what one would want all other persons to do in the same situation,[77] but that when conscience is properly formed it also takes into consideration the perspectives of other moral agents and thereby effectively represents the moral point of view. This is why Langston is able to make such a sweeping suggestion about the relevance of the dictates of one person's conscience to the lives and deliberations of others.

For Callahan, Langston, and Blustein, the extensive normative reach of conscience is justified because conscience involves moral deliberation and moral reasons that can be communicated to others. If this were not so, if one person's conscience were merely his private feelings in response to a moral issue, it is hard to see how other persons should be expected to take that individual's conscience seriously and as anything more than an expression of individual taste or preference in the moral sphere.

VI. SUMMARY

As traditionally understood, conscience involves the paradox that its judgments are, for an individual, simultaneously authoritative *and* fallible. Moreover, the fallibility of conscience does not weaken its authority, since that authority has a moral sovereignty predicated on an individual's human dignity and freedom that creates a moral imperative which compels an individual to do what she believes is right. But this authority does not mean that conscience is self-justifying or beyond questioning and reasoning. Christian theological traditions affirm both the authority and fallibility of conscience on the belief that it is both a divine endowment,

[75] Callahan, *In good conscience*, 19.
[76] Langston, *Conscience and other virtues*, 131.
[77] Ibid., 175.

enabling the apprehension of an objective moral order that God has created, and a capacity susceptible to human evil and error, requiring external standards (especially divine revelation and human reason) to correct the risk of error and inordinate subjectivity. Philosophical interpretations see the authority of conscience as arising from moral agency and the compelling relationship between moral belief and action. On such accounts, conscience is the ultimate subjective norm of individual morality because of the individual's moral responsibility to act according to the moral beliefs and assessments she takes to be true.

As a subjective norm, the exercise of conscience risks the promotion of moral individualism. As described by Charles Taylor, moral individualism can be inspired by a laudable principle of mutual self-respect that accords each person the right to develop his or her own form of life on the basis of what he or she considers to be of greatest value. But when this individualism is merely a matter of self-fulfillment, it distorts the moral ideal of authenticity by abandoning the interconnection between one's inner moral voice and any external source of moral guidance. Such individualism is self-defeating because it disregards our obligations to others and anything beyond our own desires and aspirations. By disregarding demands beyond the self, we trivialize moral decision making and fail to see that both authenticity and personal identity require a background of moral meaning against which our choices can be measured. Taylor's critique serves as a reminder that claims of conscience by themselves should not be taken as self-justifying. Instead, conscience-based claims should indicate how moral beliefs and values are related to moral positions and actions, which requires moral explanation and reasoning.

As an ultimate subjective norm, conscience is always binding, even if it is mistaken, for it represents the final and best assessment of what a person believes is right, even if that assessment might in fact be wrong. The risk of error is addressed by the Catholic tradition's emphasis on an individual's responsibility to ensure that her conscience is properly *informed* in particular situations about relevant facts, moral values, and sources of guidance. Conscience can also be misled by self-deception and rationalization. Mistakes in moral reasoning, weaknesses in moral character, and self-deception explain why conscience should never be treated as if it were beyond questioning and dialogue.

The Catholic tradition also points to a need to *form* one's conscience, so that it is habitually less likely to succumb to error. This is done through education within a moral or spiritual community that cultivates conscience through values, exemplars, narratives, and shared practices.

Whether guided by a religious or other kind of belief system, the formation of conscience entails a developmental process of integrating moral reasoning, moral emotions, and moral action. Internal motivation, a teachable spirit, and an appreciation for moral narratives are seen as vital requirements, as is an attitude of humility, which can be seen as the fitting response to the paradoxical relationship between the authority and fallibility of conscience. Humility facilitates self-scrutiny that encourages confidence without arrogance, a readiness to learn from others and to acknowledge prejudices, a willingness to modify judgments in light of further information or better insights, and an awareness of the need for an external, objective norm of morality to avoid inordinate subjectivity.

While decisions of conscience are ultimately individual, they are shaped by communities formed by social relationships. Moral communities provide socially sanctioned norms that are internalized within an individual's conscience, creating an equilibrium between the moral values of the community and the moral values of the individual. This places checks on individuals against the risk of moral self-delusion, even as it also allows individuals to challenge and sustain the reigning values of the community.

Viewed within the dynamic interplay between individuals and their moral communities, the normative reach of conscience can be seen as extending beyond the individual. When conscientious judgments are articulated as explanatory reasons that are universalizable, moral reasoning expands the relevance of one person's conscience to other persons. The reach of conscience includes other persons when reason serves as a communicative bridge from one person's conscience to another's. When social and political arrangements encourage the free expression of conscience, the content of conscience-based claims can contribute to the moral dialogue and debate of the community. Much rests on the question of the normative reach of conscience. Depending on the answer given, conscience will be seen either as something restricted to the private realm of the individual or as a source of moral assessment that is also relevant in the professional-public sphere.

6

Conscience as Integrity

I. CONSCIENCE AS INTEGRITY AND ITS RELATION TO PERSONAL UNITY AND MORAL IDENTITY

The diverse conceptions of conscience described in Chapter 4 illustrate the range of interpretations that have been attributed to a widely recognized but nevertheless controversial feature of human experience. Historical examples include conceiving of conscience as (1) a natural endowment discriminating between right and wrong, with the capacity to apply painful self-criticism and rebuke when one commits or contemplates wrongdoing (St. Paul, Butler), (2) practical reason applied to moral matters (Aquinas), (3) the apprehension of the divine judgment of one's sins (Luther, Calvin), and (4) a universal moral judge within each individual moral agent (Kant). Contemporary examples include conscience as (1) reasoned moral judgment (D'Arcy, Dineen), (2) critical self-reflection with an emotive component (Childress), (3) the cognitive power to reflect, the emotive disposition to feel, and the conative disposition to act (Broad, Langston, S. Callahan, Sulmasy, Pellegrino), (4) a cognitive and emotive capacity, qualified by a distinction between critical and uncritical conscience (Garnett), (5) the motivation to harmonize one's actions with one's knowledge and belief and thereby achieve personal integrity (Fuss, with related emphases in Duncan-Jones, McGuire, Childress), and (6) awareness of moral truth (Grisez and Shaw). Further aspects of contemporary conceptions of conscience include a dependence on truth (Ratzinger), an authority that is personal and yet generalizable (Langston), and a relation to human dignity, the pursuit of ultimate moral/spiritual meaning, and the fulfillment of moral/religious obligations (Nussbaum, Rawls). Given these diverse and multifaceted assessments that all together form a rich constellation of moral characteristics, it is appropriate now to consider how conscience is intimately related to (and often enough indistinguishable from) notions of personal unity, moral identity, and integrity.

The need for personal unity may be implicit or explicit in discussions of conscience. According to Bonhoeffer, for instance, conscience is an awareness of the need human beings have to be in union with themselves by acting in harmony with their knowledge of good and evil.[1] Conscience alerts us to inconsistencies between our understanding of what is impermissible and our failures to follow that understanding in our actions, and it identifies such inconsistencies as manifestations of personal disunity. We should always follow conscience because it "comes from a depth which lies beyond a man's own will and his own reason and it makes itself heard as the call of human existence to unity with itself" and therefore protests against doing anything that imperils this unity.[2] For Bonhoeffer, to act against one's own conscience is effectively to destroy one's own being, causing him to conclude that it is no coincidence that violations of conscience are often accompanied by attempts at suicide.[3]

The unity of the moral life in each individual is prominent in Aristotelian perspectives, in which the virtuous person is promised a certain harmony of soul that is free of conflicting desires and marked by a conscious awareness of who she is, what she wants, and what she is doing.[4] MacIntyre's description of a virtue-based life emphasizes this unity by noting how virtues, by definition, are expressed with a consistency that does not fluctuate with changes in social roles or personal circumstances. For MacIntyre, a virtue becomes intelligible only when it is a characteristic of a unitary life defined by a unifying narrative that forms an individual's life goals and thereby defines the goods that are most worth pursuing.[5] A consequence of this moral vision is that individuals are more than a mere concatenation of their various roles and decisions in life.[6]

The notion that each human life has a certain unity can also be found in John Rawls. In rejecting the possibility of identifying a single dominant vision of the good that should determine the political structures of a just society, Rawls gives moral priority to "the right" rather than "the good" on the basis of a Kantian concept of moral personality that includes the

1 Bonhoeffer, *Ethics*, 24.
2 Ibid., 242.
3 Ibid.
4 Lear, *Aristotle: the desire to understand*, 167–89.
5 MacIntyre, *After virtue*, 218.
6 MacIntyre, "Social structures and their threats to moral agency," 315.

conviction that each person has a basic unity as a human being. Having moral personality means having the individual freedom to choose one's final ends or aims. Rawls claims that the self's essential unity is a universal feature of persons that is contained in the conception of the right, and the structure of Rawls's original position itself is designed to establish the appropriate conditions for each person to fashion his or her own unity. The development and preservation of this personal unity is a guiding goal for every person's life.[7]

Closely related to the notion of personal unity is the idea of moral integrity, a concept frequently affirmed in contemporary discussions of conscience. Conceptually, moral integrity bears a close and at times indistinguishable relationship with conscience, and it has the welcome linguistic advantage of indicating the central importance of *integration* in the moral life. As will be discussed, the preservation of moral integrity involves ensuring that our moral beliefs, values, and actions are sustained within a coherent and harmonious whole that provides the basis for a sense of moral identity and moral purpose. The intimate relationship between moral integrity and conscience is illustrated by accounts that describe them in similar or parallel terms. For instance, one finds the following kinds of statements in commentaries on conscience: to act according to conscience is to act with integrity;[8] to fulfill moral or religious obligations is a matter of respecting the liberty of conscience and securing integrity;[9] and judgments of conscience are the central bases of moral integrity.[10]

In some writers there may be a subtle contrast between conscience and integrity that suggests a sequence that runs from the beginning to the end of a process of moral deliberation and action. If the function of conscience is understood to be the facilitation of moral reflection that produces moral judgments and motivates moral actions, then integrity is the moral quality that is experienced and possessed when conscience has successfully prompted a person to make his actions consistent with his beliefs and judgments. On this view, integrity would represent the outcome of conscientious living, and as such would suggest that integrity and conscience are inseparable rather than identical. This inseparability constitutes an interdependence that can be found in Fuss's conclusion

7 Rawls, *A theory of justice*, 561–63.

8 Spohn, "Conscience and moral development," 132–33.

9 Rawls, *A theory of justice*, 206.

10 Dan W. Brock, "Conscientious refusal by physicians and pharmacists: who is obligated to do what, and why?" *Theoretical Medicine and Bioethics* 29 (2008): 189.

that conscience drives us to make our actions consistent with our knowledge and beliefs and therefore has a unifying and integrating function that, when satisfied, results in a sense of integrity or wholeness.[11] Beauchamp and Childress reveal a similar assessment in their discussion of the virtues of integrity and conscientiousness when they describe conscience as a form of critical self-reflection about the morality of actions that, when ethical standards are knowingly violated, can cause a person to experience a loss of integrity.[12] Some writers see conscience as creating a sense of obligation to do that which preserves moral integrity. For instance, Garnett describes conscience as a person's authentic voice that serves as the guardian of integrity,[13] Sulmasy holds that conscience is a fundamental moral commitment to moral integrity,[14] and Pellegrino claims that "fidelity to conscience is closely identified with preservation of personal moral integrity."[15] Similarly, Wicclair believes that appeals to conscience can be interpreted as expressions of concern to preserve moral integrity,[16] and Blustein speaks of appeals to conscience as deriving from concern for integrity arising from our moral duty "to lead personally integrated lives, to bring our actions and motivations into harmony with our principles."[17] Callahan so emphasizes integration in her description of conscience that further reference to integrity seems almost redundant: conscience entails "a unified integration of thinking, feeling, and willingness to act" and "operates as a fully integrated, fully together, self-conscious activity in which no one capacity of a person acts in isolation."[18]

These examples illustrate how interrelated and overlapping integrity and conscience are, an observation that invites us to treat them as largely interchangeable labels for a single moral domain. Even so, it is worth considering a bit further the meanings that integrity carries and the descriptions it may be given. A pervasive and defining theme among commentators on integrity, and as reflected in its etymology, is wholeness. The English *integrity* originates from the Latin *integritas*, which is derived from the Latin *integer*, meaning "entire." The root meaning of *integrity*,

[11] Fuss, "Conscience," 47–48.
[12] Beauchamp and Childress, *Principles of biomedical ethics*, 44.
[13] Garnett, "Conscience and conscientiousness," 87.
[14] Sulmasy, "What is conscience and why is respect for it so important?"
[15] Pellegrino, "The physician's conscience, conscience clauses, and religious belief."
[16] M. R. Wicclair, "Conscientious objection in medicine," *Bioethics* 14 (2000): 205–27.
[17] Blustein, "Doing what the patient orders."
[18] Callahan, *In good conscience*, 15.

therefore, has to do with being whole, intact, sound, complete, and undivided (*Merriam-Webster Dictionary*).

The musical metaphor of harmony can be added to these linguistic considerations, since integrity connotes the congruous interweaving of parts into a pleasing and meaningful whole. Moral integrity indicates how the moral life aims to achieve a congruent arrangement of different parts to compose a moral identity that is internally harmonious and whole. Alfonso Gomez-Lobo uses the metaphor of harmony in his description of integrity as the opposite of hypocrisy and the presence of "the inner harmony of a human being who does not let her thoughts, attitudes, desires, emotions, utterances, and actions go asunder but brings them into fundamental consistency."[19] Jonathan Glover notes the priority Socrates placed on the need for inner moral harmony as recorded in Plato's *Gorgias.* For Socrates, true happiness required an internal peace through the possession of self-knowledge and the avoidance of self-conflict. Drawing from Socrates, Glover claims that humans need to be psychologically and morally integrated and internally at peace. Internal disharmony, suggests Glover, "involves slavery to madness, and allows the beast in man to gain control," and he quotes Socrates to stress how imperative internal harmony is: "'It would be better for me to have a musical instrument or a chorus which I was directing in discord and out of tune, better that the mass of mankind should disagree with me and contradict me than that I, a single individual, should be out of harmony with myself and contradict myself.' (*Gorgias,* 482)."[20]

Some authors identify integrity as a virtue. Pellegrino and Thomasma consider integrity the virtue that integrates "all the virtues into a whole and can prudentially judge the relative importance in each situation of principles, rules, guidelines, precepts, and the other virtues in reaching a decision to act."[21] Beauchamp and Childress describe it as a virtue with two related aspects: generally speaking it refers to "soundness, reliability, wholeness, and integration of moral character," and more narrowly it refers to "fidelity in adherence to moral norms."[22] Another perspective is offered by MacIntyre, for whom integrity is the virtue that links the countless practical ethical actions of each individual over a lifetime to the

19 Alfonso Gomez-Lobo, *Morality and the human goods: an introduction to natural law* (Washington, DC: Georgetown University Press, 2002), 23.

20 Jonathan Glover, *Humanity: a moral history of the twentieth century* (New Haven, CT: Yale University Press, 1999), 27.

21 Pellegrino and Thomasma, *The virtues in medical practice,* 127.

22 Beauchamp and Childress, *Principles of biomedical ethics,* 41–42.

end (*telos*) that defines and guides the entirety of each individual's life. For MacIntyre, the need for integrity represents the need we have as humans for our actions to make sense within an encompassing life narrative. To make this kind of sense, our actions have to be driven by a singleness of purpose that is provided by a guiding end, which provides the constancy that the virtue of integrity reflects.[23] For Wicclair, integrity may not be labeled a virtue, but it is nevertheless similar to a virtue when it is described as an integral relation between a person's core ethical values and her moral identity that requires consistency between actions and values as a matter of personal necessity.[24]

Another way of seeing how close the relationship is between conscience and integrity is to consider the adverse consequences that are believed to arise when conscience is violated and integrity is lost. When this happens, it is widely agreed that persons experience deeply negative feelings. Childress speaks of "a fundamental loss of integrity, wholeness, and harmony in the self"[25] due to a failure to follow the considered judgments of conscience. He believes that such failures arise when there is inconsistency between belief and action that leads to feelings of guilt and shame,[26] or a "bad conscience." Fuss refers to the "sense of inner failure, frustration, or guilt" that arises when one forfeits integrity by willfully choosing to disregard conscience.[27] Others describe the psychological misery,[28] loss of self-respect,[29] and effective self-betrayal[30] that ensue when conscience is ignored and integrity violated. These reactions reveal the profound psychological and spiritual import of conscience and integrity, as well as their vulnerability. And these reactions remind us of some of the reasons that liberty of conscience is taken so seriously in liberal democratic societies. We place great value on the experience of integrity when conscience is satisfied, and we express great concern about the deeply negative psychological and spiritual reactions that ensue when conscience is impeded and integrity lost.

It might be suggested that people at times find themselves in circumstances in which they are unable to uphold integrity because an action

[23] MacIntyre, *After virtue*, 203.
[24] Wicclair, "Conscientious objection in medicine."
[25] Childress, "Appeals to conscience."
[26] Childress, "Conscience and conscientious actions in the context of MCOs."
[27] Fuss, "Conscience," 43.
[28] Granrose, "The authority of conscience," 28.
[29] Garnett, "Conscience and conscientiousness," 86.
[30] Wicclair, "Conscientious objection in medicine."

plan that would fulfill all of their moral values seems unavailable. Blustein engages this problem and suggests that compromise and integrity are not necessarily mutually incompatible. He believes that integrity is fundamentally about doing one's best to live according to one's values and principles, but he also believes that there are situations in which competition among one's different moral commitments creates tension in a particular circumstance that precludes adherence to each of one of those commitments. Blustein introduces the possibility of an "integrity-preserving compromise" and argues that compromise can preserve integrity if the compromise "takes into account the whole fabric of one's relevant moral principles and values, along with the weights one gives them, and does what one judges ought to be done, all things considered."[31] In the process of such compromise, he writes, "one partially abandons or sets aside a principle or commitment, departs from a normative standpoint which one adopted before the circumstances of compromise arose and which is not completely relinquished even as the compromise is more or less reluctantly accepted."[32]

But Blustein's use of the notion of compromise is open to question, and not merely because of the superficial sense in which the idea of an "integrity-preserving compromise" sounds puzzling. If the outcome of conscientious moral deliberation genuinely preserves integrity, it would be more apt to say that the process of deliberation has led to the conclusion that a less important value ought to be superseded by a more important one, making the conclusion morally right. Such conclusions are common in the moral life, in which responsible action prioritizes one value over another, depending on an overall assessment of goals to be pursued and obligations to be fulfilled. Such conclusions represent the fulfillment of conscience and the preservation of integrity because they are based on our best moral judgments, not because they presume that every one of our particular moral values or commitments has been fulfilled in a given case. Blustein's discussion encourages us to consider how we understand and reconcile competing values that arise in the process of moral deliberation and to consider the extent to which the moral life includes grappling with what Nagel refers to as the fragmentation of value[33] or what Taylor calls the diversity of

[31] Blustein, "Doing what the patient orders."

[32] Ibid.

[33] Thomas Nagel, "The fragmentation of value," in *Knowledge, value and belief*, ed. H. Tristram Engelhardt and Daniel Callahan (Hastings-on-Hudson, NY: Institute of Society, Ethics and the Life Sciences, 1977), 279–94.

goods,[34] both of which indicate the need for practical wisdom that weighs, balances, and discerns in order to navigate and reconcile the tensions that are native to the moral landscape.

II. INTEGRITY AS A QUALITATIVELY DISTINCT VALUE, AND THE IDEA OF A PERSON'S MORAL PROJECTS

The value of preserving individual moral integrity carries important implications within a morally pluralistic society that at times struggles to reconcile individual moral freedom with political order, whether that order is based on the will of a democratic majority, the ruling of a court, or the policies of a hospital. Of special concern here are the consequentialist assumptions that may guide political decision making and conflate the many actions of diverse persons into a single causal stream defined by a single outcome that diminishes the personal significance of individual moral responsibility. Two philosophers, Charles Taylor and Bernard Williams, have addressed how this kind of consequentialist reasoning can create moral tension for individuals due to the incommensurability of individual moral integrity (compared with other goods) arising from the definitive role integrity plays in moral agency and personhood. Their contributions argue for the need to respect the irreducible significance of a person's moral integrity against pressures that might minimize or relativize its value.

In an essay entitled "The Diversity of Goods," Taylor addresses a central problem in philosophies, such as utilitarianism, that reduce and homogenize the domain of morality and thereby obscure "the qualitative distinctions we make between different actions, or feelings, or modes of life, as being in some way morally higher or lower, noble or base, admirable or contemptible."[35] Taylor argues that these qualitative distinctions are basic to moral thinking and cannot, without distortion, be removed from it. One example of a qualitative distinction is integrity.

> For some people, personal integrity is a central goal: what matters is that one's life express what one truly senses as important, admirable, noble, desirable. The temptations to be avoided here are those of conformity to established standards which are not really one's own, or of dishonesty with oneself concerning one's own convictions or affinities. The chief threat to

[34] Taylor, "The diversity of goods."
[35] Ibid., 132.

integrity is a lack of courage in the face of social demands, or in the face of what one has been brought up to see as the unthinkable.[36]

An individual has integrity to the extent that his words and actions genuinely express what he believes and values, and to that extent those words and actions have an intrinsic character that is what counts morally, rather than their consequences.[37] A consequentialist might respond by arguing that the value of personal integrity could be defended on consequentialist grounds (e.g., benefits to society), but Taylor argues that such explanations fail to explain why integrity matters to us intrinsically, apart from consequences that might flow from it. Taylor objects to any attempt to distort integrity by reducing its value to its consequences.

Williams also takes issue with utilitarianism and its failure to take integrity seriously. He objects because utilitarianism can make only superficial sense of human desire, action, and responsibility, and it fails to appreciate how one person's actions stand in relation to other persons' actions. He maintains that utilitarianism fails to recognize that "each of us is specially responsible for what he does, rather than for what other people do," and as a result it "makes integrity as a value more or less unintelligible."[38] The reason for this failure is that utilitarianism is at a loss to describe how a person's *moral projects* relate to her actions.[39] For Williams, moral projects represent the moral intentions or purposes to which a person is committed and with which he is identified and wishes to be associated. These moral projects are formed by the fundamental desires and concerns that constitute a person's moral character.[40] He argues that the negative moral feelings that arise when a person is confronted with an action that is acceptable on utilitarian terms but objectionable on nonutilitarian terms are not merely due to "self-indulgent squeamishness"; rather, these negative feelings reflect something genuine about a person's moral identity and purpose, and therefore should not be regarded as mere objects of utilitarian value. Moral feelings, argues Williams, are part of the way we relate to our world, and to dismiss these feelings on the basis of a utilitarian calculation is to act as if they exist outside of one's moral self. Such a dismissal would reflect a loss of integrity

36 Ibid., 133.
37 Ibid., 144.
38 J. J. C. Smart and Bernard Williams, *Utilitarianism: for and against* (Cambridge: Cambridge University Press, 1973), 99.
39 Ibid., 100.
40 Bernard Williams, *Moral luck* (Cambridge: Cambridge University Press, 1981), 5.

through self-alienation, not only from one's moral feelings, but also from one's moral self.[41]

Williams describes how utilitarian reasoning frames individual action within a causal nexus that is supposed to maximize utility to increase the satisfaction (happiness) of all parties involved. In this causal nexus, the moral projects of all parties are mixed together in one heterogeneous aggregation. The individual moral agent is supposed, according to utilitarian thinking, to act in such a way that there will be a greater sum total of satisfaction for all concerned. However, the problem is that the outcome of a utilitarian calculation may represent a decision that conflicts with the moral project of the individual moral agent in question. At this point, the challenge is not merely one of balancing or incorporating diverse interests, for when an individual's moral project is at stake, it is not adequate to suggest that this project be considered as just one interest or satisfaction among many others. Moral projects are those commitments around which people build their lives and on which they stake their identities, and as a result these projects are not to be treated as if they are amenable to mixture within, and direction by, the causal nexus that is determined by other projects, other interests, and other actions.[42] Williams provides a vivid summary of why it is unacceptable to expect the individual to resign his moral project to the dictates of the surrounding causal nexus:

> It is absurd to demand of such a man, when the sums come in from the utility network which the projects of others have in part determined, that he should just step aside from his own project and decision and acknowledge the decision which utilitarian calculation requires. It is to alienate him in a real sense from his actions and the source of his action in his convictions. It is to make him into a channel between the input of everyone's projects, including his own, and an output of optimific decision; but this is to neglect the extent to which his actions and his decisions have to be seen as the actions and decisions which flow from the projects and attitudes with which he is most closely identified. It is thus, in the most literal sense, an attack on his integrity.[43]

Williams also faults utilitarianism for distorting individual moral agency (with which integrity is so closely associated), objecting to the way it effectively denies the separateness of persons. By maximizing total or average utility, utilitarianism agglomerates satisfactions in a way that is indifferent

41 Smart and Williams, *Utilitarianism*, 103–104.
42 Ibid., 115–16.
43 Ibid., 116–17.

to the separateness of the persons who have those satisfactions. A second area of concern pertains to the relationship between moral agency and states of affairs. Williams argues that in utilitarianism the basic bearer of value is not a person (or set of differentiated persons) but a state of affairs, for it does not matter *who* produces (or contributes to producing) a state of affairs, but only *that* a certain state of affairs exists.[44] A third area of concern is the possibility that those who insist on preserving their own integrity are guilty of moral self-indulgence – as illustrated, according to some, by a person's refusing to participate in an objectionable action, while acknowledging that the action will predictably take place nevertheless because others will be willing to participate. Critics claim that this supposed moral self-indulgence represents a possessive attitude toward one's own virtue[45] and that the "other-concern" advocated by utilitarianism is here opposed to a "self-concern" prompted by individual integrity. Williams responds to this critique by arguing that it fails to appreciate that integrity (unlike other virtues) does not have a characteristic thought or action associated with it, a feature that makes it seem as though integrity is focused on oneself. Rather, the focus of integrity is on the projects a person cares most about, and it is in pursuing those projects that she displays her integrity.[46]

I will return to concerns related to moral self-indulgence later in this chapter, when considering the suggestion that one should sometimes be willing to sacrifice one's conscience in the service of another person's important interests. At this point, however, to anticipate Chapter 9, it should be noted how important individual moral agency is for conscientious objection and conscientious practice, since the practice of medicine is full of opportunities for physicians and other health care professionals to participate (or decline to participate) in the causal nexus of decision making in which they find themselves. These situations can involve physicians with patients, colleagues, health care teams, practices, hospitals, health systems, insurers, or governments. They may include treating, assisting, advising, informing, or referring, and in each case they may raise questions for the physician about participating in a decision, process, or action that is foreign to his own moral projects. Questions about participation may be minimized by persons adopting a consequentialist view predicated on outcomes. But such questions will be taken seriously by

44 Williams, *Moral luck*, 3–4.
45 Ibid., 40.
46 Ibid., 49.

those who share the concerns of Taylor and Williams, because they will see the preservation of integrity as an irreducible value that should never be taken as merely one interest among others within an overriding utilitarian calculation that proposes to maximize satisfactions.

III. THE IMPLAUSIBILITY OF DIVIDING CONSCIENCE OR INTEGRITY INTO PERSONAL AND PROFESSIONAL PARTS

Given what has been said about conscience and integrity – regarding their relation to personal unity, moral identity, and moral projects – it may be surprising that there are some who believe a person's conscience or integrity[47] can be divided into personal and professional domains. Nevertheless, such a proposed divisibility can be found in recent literature on the status of conscientious objection by health care professionals, and it suggests that there are at least two prevailing conceptions regarding conscience or integrity with regard to their unitary or divisible status. On the one hand, there are those who see conscience or integrity as essentially integrated and indivisible, involving the whole person and the entire moral self. On the other hand, there are those who see conscience or integrity as having the capacity for division, compartmentalization, or, we might even say, dis-integration. Far from being merely a theoretical consideration, the question about the unitary or divisible status of conscience or integrity has very practical implications. The question bears not only on the extent to which medical professionals should be allowed to act according to conscience or integrity, but also on how we should understand the moral origins of the beliefs and values that sustain the ethics, professionalism, and humanism that motivate and guide the practices of medical professionals.

One of the ways in which some persons may propose to divide the domain of conscience is by consigning conscience to the realm of the "personal" and thereby separating it from the realm of the "professional." Such a designation is suggested, at least in part, in the policy statement on conscientious refusal published by the American College of Obstetricians

[47] I refer to conscience *or* integrity to cover references to both, because I favor treating them as largely interchangeable labels for a single moral domain and because the authors to be discussed in this section tend to frame their remarks either in terms of conscience or in terms of integrity.

and Gynecologists (ACOG).[48] This document adopts a definition of conscience as a "private, constant, ethically attuned part of the human character" and views a conflict of conscience as a "personal moral problem" such that to act against one's conscience would be to risk harming one's "personal wholeness or identity." The authors of this document appreciate that conscience involves "a provider's right to protect his or her moral integrity," and they acknowledge that "personal conscience" has "a critical and useful place in the practice of medicine." They add, moreover, that "[i]n many cases, [personal conscience] can foster thoughtful, effective, and humane care." However, these authors also believe that conscience poses a problem because it "may conflict with professional and ethical standards and result in inefficiency, adverse outcomes, violation of patients' rights, and erosion of trust if, for example, one's conscience limits the information or care provided to a patient."

By juxtaposing "personal conscience" and "professional and ethical standards," these authors risk implying that the "personal" moral realm is somehow distinct from, and not in a contributing relationship with, the "professional" moral realm and its ethical standards. In an attempt to reconcile claims that may arise from these competing realms, they perceive the need for "a balance between respect for conscience and other important values" in order to facilitate "the ethical practice of medicine." More specifically, the authors believe that "respect for conscience must be weighed against respect for particular social values" and that even "when a provider's moral integrity is truly at stake, there are clearly limits to the degree to which appeals to conscience may justifiably guide decision making." Accordingly, they attempt to justify the subordination of conscience on two grounds. First, they claim that conscience is "only a prima facie value, which means it can and should be overridden in the interest of other moral obligations that outweigh it in a given circumstance." Second, they claim that "[p]rofessional ethics requires that health [*sic*] be delivered in a way that is respectful of patient autonomy, timely and effective, evidence based, and nondiscriminatory." The authors thereby invoke the principle of respect for patient autonomy as a moral principle that is superior to the protection of conscience – notwithstanding that respect for autonomy is itself a value that is usually understood in prima facie, not absolute, terms in biomedical ethics.[49]

48 ACOG, Committee on Ethics, "The limits of conscientious refusal in reproductive medicine (ACOG committee opinion no. 385)," *Obstetrics and Gynecology* 110 (2007): 1203–1208.

49 Beauchamp and Childress, *Principles of biomedical ethics*.

As further evidence of the ACOG statement's tendency to assign conscience to the personal realm, the authors refer to the need to ensure that the "provider's personal interests" yield to his "professional responsibilities to patients," going so far as to say that physicians "are bound by special *fiduciary duties*, which oblige physicians to act in good faith to protect patients' health – particularly to the extent that patients' health interests conflict with physicians' personal or self-interest." These remarks give the impression that conscience is ultimately private, personal, self-oriented, and possibly even self-serving – a conceptualization that stands in stark contrast to conscience as the expression of moral integrity, wholeness of personality, and the individual's guide and motivation for all moral actions, including those focused altruistically on the patient's good.

It is true that in places the ACOG statement treats conscience in relationship with integrity, such as when it discusses the basis of a physician's opposition to actions imposed by an external authority that would harm or detract from patients' interests. In this case the authors acknowledge connections between conscience, integrity, goals of medicine, and fiduciary obligations to patients. But generally speaking, their remarks do not portray conscience as an entity that includes moral reasoning, and they do not consistently correlate conscience with the characteristics of integrity. Instead, the authors' preponderant tendency is apparently to treat conscience as a private, personal entity that may be more concerned with a physician's own interests than with moral beliefs and values that are generally relevant and necessary for addressing professional questions about the definition of health, the goals of medicine, and the extent of a physician's fiduciary obligation to respect expressions of patient self-determination.

Another example of a policy statement that consigns conscience to the personal realm can be found in the American Academy of Pediatrics (AAP) statement on conscientious refusals, which relies centrally on a proposed distinction between professional and nonprofessional domains and the need for their separation and prioritization. The AAP statement draws this distinction by stating that those who claim "that the exercise of conscience is integral to being a professional" are guilty of confusing "professional and nonprofessional commitments."[50] Moreover, the writers of the AAP policy add an epistemological gloss to this distinction by asserting that "conscientious objections are typically based not on medical

[50] AAP, Committee on Bioethics, "Policy statement: physician refusal to provide information or treatment on the basis of claims of conscience," *Pediatrics* 124 (2009): 1689–93.

knowledge but on moral, religious, or political beliefs," thereby attributing knowledge to the professional domain, and belief to the nonprofessional domain. As discussed in Chapter 1, the pluralism that surrounds our notions of health, disease, and the goals of medicine reveals the degree to which these notions and goals are normatively laden and resist easy distinction between professional knowledge and personal belief.

The proposal that conscience should be restricted largely to the realm of a professional's private life can also be found in the writings of some commentators in medical journals. Some writers claim a distinction between private conscience and public acts, maintaining that because of their public responsibility to fulfill a unique social role, physicians should not be entitled to an unqualified right of conscience, and sincere claims of conscience should not necessarily be respected if the actions directed by those claims significantly and negatively affect patients.[51] Others contrast the personal domain of conscience with the public domain of patient care and propose a personal–public dichotomy in which personal (and specifically religious) beliefs are viewed as illegitimate reasons for actions that conflict with the preferences of patients regarding legally available services.[52] Another writer claims that "values and conscience have different roles in public and private life" and as such "should not influence the care an individual doctor offers to his or her patient."[53] In this last case, conscience is deemed an inappropriate source of moral authority for the physician's work because it is viewed as serving the physician's interest and contradicting the injunction that, as public servants, physicians "must act in the public interest, not their own."[54] This view drives a sharp wedge between the private and the public, restricting the physician's values and conscience to private life and making them of questionable relevance to the public domain of patient care.

Sometimes authors explicitly claim that a person's conscience or integrity can be divided. They invoke such a claim to suggest that a line be drawn between the personal and the professional domains of a health care professional's life. One example of this division arises in a discussion

[51] Eva LaFollette and Hugh LaFollette, "Private conscience, public acts," *Journal of Medical Ethics* 33 (2007): 249–54.

[52] Julie Cantor and Ken Baum, "The limits of conscientious objection: may pharmacists refuse to fill prescriptions for emergency contraception?" *New England Journal of Medicine* 351 (2004): 2008–12.

[53] Julian Savulescu, "Conscientious objection in medicine," *British Medical Journal* 332 (2006): 294–97.

[54] Ibid.

of the conditions under which induced abortion and feticide are justifiable.[55] To support the claim that physicians who object to abortion still have an obligation to provide information about abortion and referral to abortion services, the authors of this discussion make conscience divisible by introducing a distinction between "professional conscience" and "individual conscience." Professional conscience, they say, "is shaped by autonomy-based and beneficence-based obligations of the obstetrician to the pregnant and fetal patients" and is based on "professional medical ethics." Individual conscience, they say, appeals "to sources of morality other than professional medical ethics, such as personal experience, family upbringing, and religion." These authors take individual conscience seriously, recognizing that a physician's "individual moral convictions, values, and beliefs" may mean that "some pregnant women cannot become or continue to be patients of a particular physician." But these authors believe that physicians who are unable to care for certain patients (on the basis of individual conscience) still have an obligation to inform and refer (on the basis of professional conscience), and to that extent they grant professional conscience the prerogative to constrain individual conscience. It appears the authors are attempting to resolve tensions arising from conscientious objection by separating conscience into two parts. In doing so, they appear to assign the moral interests of the patient to professional conscience and the moral interests of the physician to individual conscience.

There are also authors who describe integrity as divisible. One of these is Martin Benjamin, who bases this divisibility on the idea that perspectives on integrity can be internal or external. Benjamin defines integrity as consisting of three elements that together form a person's moral identity: "(1) a reasonably coherent and relatively stable set of highly cherished values and principles; (2) verbal behavior expressing these values and principles; and (3) conduct embodying one's values and principles and consistent with what one says."[56] He then suggests that integrity can be viewed either internally (from the point of view of the person) or externally (from the point of view of others). Internally, integrity provides the basis for a life that is unified and whole; externally, integrity provides the basis for relationships marked by trust, friendship, and love. The external

[55] Frank A. Chervenak and Laurence B. McCullough, "An ethically justified practical approach to offering, recommending, performing, and referring for induced abortion and feticide," *American Journal of Obstetrics and Gynecology* 201 (2009): 560.e1–6.

[56] Martin Benjamin, *Splitting the difference: compromise and integrity in ethics and politics* (Lawrence: University Press of Kansas, 1990), 51.

perspective represents a framework of value that arises from the expectations an individual experiences in her social roles, expectations that may stand in opposition to the individual's values and principles.

In response to Benjamin's proposal, we can ask whether it is helpful to expand the boundaries of integrity so that it encompasses values external to, and potentially in conflict with, the individual's own moral commitments. By expanding integrity to such an extent, we abandon a unified sense of moral integration in which competing values are prioritized and owned by the individual who responsibly performs the work of that integration. One wonders whether Benjamin's proposal for a two-perspective integrity reflects an interest in identifying a concept of integrity capable of promoting "internal and external compromise."[57] This possibility is worth considering, in light of Benjamin's expressed skepticism about the possibility of perfect integrity, his preference for a complex conception of integrity that both supports a notion of personal identity and acknowledges the need for mutual accommodation, and his willingness to abandon "the image of integrity as the perfectly interlocking pieces of a completed puzzle."[58]

Other authors who espouse the divisibility of integrity refer to "personal" integrity and "clinician" integrity.[59] They speak of personal integrity as deriving from personal values, and professional integrity as deriving from "the values, rights, and obligations that attend to being a clinician." They also speak of "the clinician's own moral agency" based on rights and interests, "some of which derive from their status as medical professionals." Whereas some authors locate both beneficence-based *and* autonomy-based concerns for the patient in professional conscience,[60] these authors separate beneficence-based concerns from those that are autonomy-based and locate beneficence-based concerns in clinician integrity when conflicts arise between beneficence and patient autonomy. The portrayal of integrity by these authors is notable not only for its proposed divisibility, but also for its giving further cause to wonder how one is supposed to decide which moral values and commitments fall into the category of "professional" when integrity or conscience is thought to be divisible.

57 Ibid., 59.
58 Ibid., 72.
59 John Lantos, Ann Marie Matlock, and David Wendler, "Clinician integrity and limits to patient autonomy," *JAMA* 305 (2011): 495–99.
60 Chervenak and McCullough, "An ethically justified practical approach to offering, recommending, performing, and referring for induced abortion and feticide."

For those who believe in such divisibility, it seems that the decision about which moral values will be considered "professional" will correlate with beliefs about which values professionals can legitimately rely on to justify decisions and actions that may significantly affect the lives of patients. Beliefs and values that are considered legitimate for this purpose will presumably be labeled "professional," and those considered illegitimate, "personal." But attempts to mark off the boundaries of such a distinction will, I believe, encounter insurmountable challenges, and not only because of the moral pluralism of medicine and society. More immediate is the concern that the beliefs and values constituting a person's integrity are so foundational, interlocking, and permeating that they transcend division and resist compartmentalization. For this reason, I do not believe that conscience or integrity is amenable to division, a position that will be elaborated later. For now, suffice it to say that the *interpersonal* tension which the dividers of conscience or integrity are apparently attempting to resolve can more appropriately be addressed if conscience or integrity is accepted as the means by which a person's moral beliefs and values are held together and by which *competing obligations* are integrated, even if there are *intrapersonal* tensions within that integration.

The preceding proposals that would divide conscience or integrity are drawn from a health care context in which professionals experience tension or conflict between the moral beliefs and values they bring to their professional activities as individuals and the social expectations that may be associated with their professional roles. Such tensions and conflicts are not restricted to health care, of course, and a discussion of the general phenomenon at issue can be found in the work of Michael Walzer, who portrays the self as an entity inherently divided by the plurality of its interests, roles, and identities.

In *Thick and Thin*, Walzer describes the self as divided among its interests and roles (citizen, parent, worker or professional or merchant, teacher or student, doctor or patient), its identities (family, nation, religion, gender, political commitment), and its ideals, principles, and values. This heterogeneity makes the self a complex entity that reflects the complexity of the social world.[61] Notably, Walzer includes conscience as part of the self that is divided and plural. He pictures conscience as a gathering of vocal critics "speaking for different values, representing different roles and identities"

[61] Michael Walzer, *Thick and thin: moral argument at home and abroad* (Notre Dame, IN: University of Notre Dame Press, 1994), 85.

that "*are me.*"[62] Self and conscience are seen as personally and socially constructed, the influence of the latter implying that persons will share divergent interpretations of the meaning of the moral knowledge that conscience provides, making conscience itself divided.[63]

Notwithstanding these fundamental divisions, Walzer suggests there is still a self that is worthy of the name, a self that is divided but not utterly fragmented:

> I can be strong and consistent in this role or identity and then in that one – much as a democratic state, despite fierce and on-going political controversy, can pursue a particular set of policies and then a different set. Without a coherent public, social criticism loses its point; without a coherent self, an ego, a *me*, the point of self-criticism is similarly lost. The picture of the self that I want to defend is *ordered*, even if the order is also, as we will see, always subject to change. I can think of myself as a confabulation of critics only if I am somehow at the center of the confabulation: not quite in charge of all the critics but their only listener and answerer, ready to say yes or no (or maybe) to each of them. There is no linearity, then, and no hierarchy. The order of the self is better imagined as a thickly populated circle, with me in the center surrounded by my self-critics who stand at different temporal and spatial removes (but don't necessarily stand still). Insofar as I am receptive to criticism, ready for (a little) castigation, I try to draw some of the critics closer, so that I am more immediately aware of their criticism; or I simply incorporate them, so that they become my intimate worriers, and I become a worried self.... My larger self, my worried self, is constituted and self-constituted by the sum of them all. I am the whole circle and also its embattled center.[64]

It is a vivid and engaging picture Walzer sketches, but it does not explain how the self is supposed to have a definable center that holds its contrasting parts together and establishes its own boundaries. There is a need for something more determinate and more grounded than his pluralistic self implies, if that self is to be more than a mere conglomeration of diverse interests, identities, and values. Walzer's self seems to be more a reflection of pluralistic society than a representation of individual moral freedom that expresses a person's identity as defined by a coherence of moral commitments that can provide guidance amid the diverse values that may exist inside and outside the self. A self needs what a political analogy like Walzer's suggests it ought to have: the personal equivalent of a constitution that expresses the fundamental values, structures, and procedures

[62] Ibid., 96.
[63] Ibid., 97.
[64] Ibid., 98–99.

that provide a coherent basis for laws, the interpretation of laws, the direction of policies, and the resolution of conflicts. Walzer's analogy invites us to ask where, in his divided self, we are to find the personal core element that plays the role of a guiding constitution. His account provides no answer to this question. Instead, he contrasts the "divided self" with the "dominated self" (the religious or political fanatic), who suffers from identifying wholeheartedly with a single all-powerful internal voice,[65] implying that a unifying basis or motivation for a singleness of purpose would be a social liability, not a moral virtue.

Walzer appears to portray a self without an internal basis for moral orientation and direction, a self that reflects the image of a diverse, democratic society, minus a guiding constitution. One wonders whether the purpose of his portrayal is to support a socially constructed view of the self that provides a congenial correspondence between a pluralistic society and a pluralistic self. Such a view of the self would seem to consign persons to lives that are not only intractably morally conflicted, but also morally directionless – like a state lacking both a constitution and leadership. What Walzer's account lacks is a self with an identity marked by core moral beliefs and values that provide the means for intentionally engaging and navigating the moral landscape.

IV. UNITING THE PERSONAL AND THE PROFESSIONAL IN AN UNDIVIDED SELF

In contrast to authors who suggest that conscience or integrity may be divided, there are those who see in moral agency a unified whole that simply does not admit of such divisions. In the health care context, Pellegrino serves as an example, able as he is to distinguish two dimensions of conscience while still arguing for their inseparability.[66] For Pellegrino, professional conscience pertains to the moral duties of the physician–patient relationship and the moral obligation to practice scientifically competent and humane medicine. Personal conscience reflects the physician's own moral beliefs (spiritual, philosophical, cultural, or ethnic) and speaks to the way a physician values human life and its implications. But Pellegrino insists that physicians cannot separate their professional from their personal lives, which would be to impose "a psychological schism that violates the

65 Ibid., 99.
66 Pellegrino, "The physician's conscience, conscience clauses, and religious belief."

integrity of the person as a unity of body, soul, and psyche."[67] Blustein similarly emphasizes the moral imperative of conscience to resist moral conflicts that threaten to inflict inner divisions that would damage the physician's integrity.[68]

With respect to individuals in society in general, MacIntyre has been one of the most notable critics of those who would in any manner attempt to make the self, or any of its essential aspects, divisible. He gives this issue considerable attention in *After Virtue*, arguing that "modernity partitions each human life into a variety of segments, each with its own norms and modes of behavior," such that "work is divided from leisure, private life from public, the corporate from the personal."[69] He sees this tendency as resulting from an atomistic view of human action and a willingness to divide a person from his social role. The willingness to partition the self from its roles stands in stark opposition to an Aristotelian understanding of virtue in which character traits apply to all parts of a person's life. The reason for this Aristotelian view arises from the belief that a virtue, if a person possesses it, has a unity in that person's life and that unity is intelligible only as a characteristic of a single life that can be understood and evaluated only as a whole.[70] For MacIntyre, a human life is characterized by a unified narrative anchored in an undivided concept of the self.

In another work, MacIntyre addresses the problem of the divided self in terms of compartmentalization.[71] Different spheres of social activity, he says, have distinct role structures and governing norms that create a compartmentalizing effect. Within each sphere, individuals are inclined to conform to the requirements imposed on their roles and, in consequence, arc deprived of the ability to step back from their roles in order "to scrutinize themselves and the structure of their society from some external standpoint with any practical effect."[72] Not only does this willingness to adopt the role imposed by a particular sphere of activity diminish an individual's capacity for critical reflection, it also divides the self. A compartmentalized self is a divided self, and therefore lacks constancy and integrity "because its allegiance to this or that set of standards is always temporary and context-bound."[73] For MacIntyre, the virtue of

[67] Ibid.
[68] Blustein, "Doing what the patient orders."
[69] MacIntyre, *After virtue*, 204.
[70] Ibid., 205.
[71] MacIntyre, "Social structures and their threats to moral agency," 321–26.
[72] Ibid.
[73] Ibid.

integrity is essential for moral agency, and to have it "is to refuse to be, to have educated oneself so that one is no longer able to be, one kind of person in one social context, while quite another in other contexts. It is to have set inflexible limits to one's adaptability to the roles that one may be called upon to play."[74] Closely related to integrity is another essential virtue, constancy, which enables people to pursue their moral goals over extended periods of time without allowing changing circumstances or contexts to distract from their moral commitments. For MacIntyre, these two virtues together allow a person to maintain focus on her moral purposes and preserve her moral character regardless of the different roles in society she is called to play.[75]

In the health care context, MacIntyre's concerns about compartmentalization are probably best represented in literature that deals with the problem of "moral distress." And given the degree to which professional activity is embedded within highly developed and often hierarchical role expectations, it is not surprising that this literature receives prominent contributions from nursing professionals, who note the ways in which a willingness to compromise one's conscience or integrity can deleteriously alter and compartmentalize oneself.[76] Such concerns are reflected in the Code of Ethics of the American Nurses Association when it describes the significance of the wholeness of personal character, the need to integrate personal and professional values, and the importance of preserving individual integrity.[77] Commentators from non-health-care disciplines also speak of the seriousness of the problem of compartmentalization. For instance, one author notes that the legal profession carries a secularized conception of the professional role that can result in "divisions of the self" in lawyers who feel compelled to separate their professional work from their religious beliefs and values.[78]

Returning to MacIntyre, it is important to note another feature of his critique of compartmentalization, and that is the negative impact a divided self can have on the potential for self-reflection and self-criticism. MacIntyre incisively argues that a self that is willing to be divided is deprived of the struggle that comes with moral conflict. Compartmentalization

74 Ibid.

75 Ibid.

76 Joan McCarthy and Rick Deady, "Moral Distress Reconsidered," *Nursing Ethics* 15, no. 2 (2008): 254–62.

77 ANA, "American Nurses Association Code of Ethics," 2001.

78 Martha Minow, "On being a religious professional: the religious turn in professional ethics," *University of Pennsylvania Law Review* 150 (2001): 687.

avoids this struggle by separating sources of conflict instead of allowing them to come into contact and create tension. A willingness to forgo the struggle of moral conflict results in a loss for a moral practice such as medicine, a practice that needs professionals who are capable of critical reflection and independent judgment to assess clinical practices and the institutional structures and social policies that guide them. Critical reflection of this kind expresses a responsible and candid approach to moral conflict that takes on the hard work of trying to resolve tensions created by competing interests or values.

Another philosopher who has written extensively about the moral meaning and implications of personal identity is Charles Taylor. His insights in *Sources of the Self*, which relate directly to conceptions of conscience and integrity that are indivisible, are based on an understanding of the intimate relationship between personal identity and moral meaning, and the nature and inescapability of moral frameworks.[79] His analysis begins with an examination of the phenomenology of our deepest moral intuitions, viewing these as our mode of access to the ontological realm in which moral claims can be sifted.[80] They are like instincts, but they also involve claims about the nature and status of human beings, which shows that a moral reaction is an assent to a given ontological perspective of what it means to be human. Though a strand of modern naturalism attempts to declare this ontological feature of our moral reactions irrelevant, the separation is not possible. The way in which we think and reason about morality presupposes that our moral reactions "are not only 'gut' feelings but also implicit acknowledgements of claims concerning their objects."[81]

Taylor observes that our moral frameworks require articulation when we are asked to describe or defend our moral reactions as right. This articulation makes explicit the moral backgrounds that routinely remain implicit in the normal course of human affairs (e.g., differences between religious and secular backgrounds are rarely disclosed, except perhaps in particularly contentious matters like abortion). Though in the context of modern naturalist sentiments the question of frameworks would be considered a pseudo-question, Taylor believes that these frameworks allow us to make sense of our lives spiritually,[82] and they do so by providing the grounds for a crucial set of qualitative distinctions. "To think, feel,

79 Charles Taylor, *Sources of the self* (Cambridge, MA: Harvard University Press, 1989), 1–52.
80 Ibid., 8.
81 Ibid., 7.
82 Ibid., 17.

judge within such a framework is to function with the sense that some action, or mode of life, or mode of feeling is incomparably higher than the others which are more readily available to us."[83] That which is incomparably higher refers to those ends or goods that are incommensurable and by which we measure the worth of our lives and endeavors. The incomparability of these goods allows for "strong evaluation" of our responses because these goods are independent of our own desires, inclinations, or choices, and they represent standards by which these are judged.[84] Frameworks are therefore "qualitative discriminations of the incomparably higher."[85] They articulate the moral backgrounds that explain and justify our moral judgments, and they inform what Taylor identifies as the three axes of moral thinking: (1) our sense of respect and obligation to others; (2) our understanding of what constitutes a full life (a life worth living); and (3) a range of notions about dignity.[86]

Taylor maintains that the naturalist temper attempts to deny frameworks altogether by supposing that all qualitative distinctions can be reduced to a quantitative scale, as typified by the reductionism of classical utilitarianism. "The aim of this philosophy was precisely to reject all qualitative distinctions and to construe all human goals as on the same footing, susceptible therefore of common quantification and calculation according to some common 'currency'."[87] But frameworks are not optional, argues Taylor, because they allow us to make sense of our lives, and to deny them would be to deny our personhood. "My identity is defined by the commitments and identifications which provide the frame or horizon within which I can try to determine from case to case what is good, or valuable, or what ought to be done, or what I endorse or oppose. In other words, it is the horizon within which I am capable of taking a stand."[88] Without such frameworks, there is a loss of moral orientation that can define the moral landscape, establish our position within that landscape, and inform us that we are moving either toward or away from the moral good that is of fundamental value to us.[89] The pursuit of what is good is therefore understood as an unfolding narrative or, à la MacIntyre, a quest.[90]

[83] Ibid., 19.
[84] Ibid., 20.
[85] Ibid., 26.
[86] Ibid., 15.
[87] Ibid., 22–23.
[88] Ibid., 27.
[89] Ibid., 41–42.
[90] Ibid., 45–48.

Another important feature of Taylor's analysis involves the role that *hypergoods* play within our moral frameworks and how these hypergoods provide a striking alternative to Walzer's view of a divided self. Hypergoods are higher-order goods that provide the standpoint from which a person judges all other goods and that provide the landmarks by which a person determines the direction of his life in order to be oriented to the highest good that is essential for her identity.[91] Various goods may serve as hypergoods, including justice, benevolence, universal and equal respect for all persons, or the love of God.[92] Taylor acknowledges that we may be motivated by a multiplicity of goods, but he contends that one good can be highest and thereby serve as a hypergood that not only provides a basis for adjudicating among lesser goods, but also has the potential to give a person "a sense of wholeness, of fullness of being as a person or self, that nothing else can."[93] But Taylor notes that hypergoods are also a source of tension, since ethical outlooks organized around them are inherently in competition and cause moral dilemmas as one tries to reconcile their respective goods. This is seen, for example, in the contrast between classical utilitarianism and Kantian deontology, each reducing the good to one dimension that stands in tension with the other. There is a tendency among reductionist theories to avoid such tensions by neglecting the values that compete against the theory or value of choice. Taylor believes that because those who adopt moral perspectives based on a single rational criterion are incapable of handling conflicts between hypergoods, they flatten a range of hypergoods into a single dimension and thereby distort the true range of value that diverse hypergoods represent. Taylor believes that a reconciliation between such hypergoods is possible but that it requires that we first recognize the hypergoods we live by in their full range.[94]

In their portrayal of moral experience and identity, MacIntyre and Taylor offer a view of the moral life that is comprehensive and fully integrated. I take his view to be accurate and the basis for justifying a strong notion of moral integrity that firmly resists suggestions about the divisibility of conscience or integrity into personal and professional domains. This perspective reflects the conviction that we are never really able, as moral persons, to detach ourselves from the primary sources of our moral energy and identity. To require detachment from our moral frameworks – what

[91] Ibid., 62–63.
[92] Ibid., 63–67.
[93] Ibid., 63.
[94] Ibid., 107.

Rawls called comprehensive doctrines – would be to invite moral disorientation. It would be to forget who we are and where we are in the moral landscape. Such an approach to the moral life is simply not available to us so long as we expect to sustain our capacity to make authentic moral choices that preserve our moral identities and provide moral orientation. In the context of medical practice and ethics, the perspective offered by MacIntyre and Taylor implies that physicians and other health care professionals should not be viewed as persons who can split their moral selves along some supposed line of demarcation that separates the personal from the professional. Instead, it should be recognized that their individual moral frameworks – not merely their acquired professional standards – are constitutive of their identities and essential to the moral meaning of their lives.

V. THE IMPLAUSIBILITY OF SACRIFICING ONE'S CONSCIENCE OR INTEGRITY FOR ANOTHER'S SAKE

Another way to discuss the undivided character of conscience or integrity arises in response to the suggestion, occasionally encountered, that persons at times may need to sacrifice their consciences in order to fulfill their moral responsibilities. The idea of a physician sacrificing her conscience for the sake of a patient is implied, for instance, when conscience is seen as an expression of self-interest, in contrast to an attitude of selflessness that focuses on the patient's welfare. Such an attitude may be operative in the statement, for example, that health care providers "should cast off the cloak of conscience when patients' needs demand it."[95] Attempts to describe conscience in self-centered terms invite us to consider whether sacrificing one's conscience for another person's sake is consistent with understanding conscience as integrity.

Granrose addresses this question by asking whether there are times when a person is "morally obligated to disobey his conscience, to sacrifice his (mental) health for the sake of others" in a way that parallels a person's decision to sacrifice her physical life for the sake of others.[96] He wrestles with this question because he is uneasy with the conclusion that there should be no limits to the individual exercise of conscience and that the interests of others (or society) should always yield to the conscience-driven actions of the individual. But he also admits to feeling "that there

[95] J. D. Cantor, "Conscientious objection gone awry: restoring selfless professionalism in medicine," *New England Journal of Medicine* 360 (2009): 1484–85.

[96] Granrose, "The authority of conscience," 228–29.

is something repugnant about compelling someone to do something which he has conscientiously concluded to be immoral."[97] Relying on John Stuart Mill's defense of the merits of individual freedom, Granrose concludes that a person should always follow her conscience – though he also believes that society may at times be justified in restraining the actions of individuals even when those actions are motivated by conscience.

Bonhoeffer assesses this question in a discussion of how a person may incur moral guilt by disobeying a moral principle in order to fulfill his moral responsibility. He uses Kant's discussion of truthfulness to explain what is occurring when, for instance, a man refuses to answer honestly to the inquiry of a murderer who breaks into the man's house to see if the man's friend (who is being pursued by the murderer) has taken refuge there. Bonhoeffer believes that Kant's conclusion to this moral dilemma (that the man must give an honest yes if the friend is in his house) is morally grotesque, because "in such a case self-righteousness of conscience has become outrageous presumption and blocks the path of responsible action."[98] He explains further: "If I refuse to incur guilt against the principle of truthfulness for the sake of my friend, if I refuse to tell a robust lie for the sake of my friend . . . if, in other words, I refuse to bear guilt for charity's sake, then my action is in contradiction to my responsibility."[99]

In these remarks Bonhoeffer is not suggesting that "responsible action" poses a threat to conscience. He maintains that accepting moral responsibility that also incurs guilt (because a moral principle such as truthfulness has been broken) must never destroy the personal unity of the ego that is at the core of conscience, for if that unity were destroyed, then this ego would no longer have the capacity to assume responsibility. Bonhoeffer here points to the self-defeating nature of the suggestion that moral responsibility may require sacrificing conscience, for conscience is fundamentally related to the preconditions of moral responsibility. That is why there are limits, according to Bonhoeffer, to the extent of moral guilt that can be incurred in the pursuit of responsible action, and those limits are defined "by the requirement of the man's unity with himself, that is to say, by his carrying power."[100] If the moral unity of a person is not preserved, then that person's moral agency and responsibility are diminished or destroyed.

97 Ibid., 232.
98 Bonhoeffer, *Ethics*, 245.
99 Ibid.
100 Ibid., 246.

There is a similarity, I think, between Bonhoeffer's remarks and the way Childress and Nagel emphasize the basic incoherence of the idea that conscience can be responsibly sacrificed in the course of fulfilling one's moral responsibility.[101] I believe they correctly maintain that conscience and integrity are fulfilled, not sacrificed, when an individual determines that a course of action is morally justified and therefore should be pursued, even when that means that an important moral commitment of lesser value must yield to one of greater value. The existence of such competing commitments amid apparently insoluble conflicts may be regrettable. And such conflicts may rightly disturb one's peace of mind, due to the sadness that comes from experiencing the fallibility of human affairs and circumstances and our limited means to improve them. But peace of mind, in this sense, is not the same as the preservation of conscience and integrity, which in the end have to do with knowing that we are acting on our best moral judgments and deepest moral convictions, all things considered. There can be personal costs to morally responsible action, even when conscience and integrity are preserved.

VI. SUMMARY

There is a relationship between conscience and the need for unity in the moral life that explains why conscience is often and appropriately viewed as moral integrity. Integrity captures the idea that conscience fundamentally involves a unifying integration of moral beliefs, values, and actions. Efforts to define moral integrity rely on notions of wholeness, completeness, and harmony. Integrity may also be viewed as a virtue that binds all other virtues into a whole, integrates moral character, or links the ethical actions of a lifetime to the end (*telos*) that guides an individual life. The connotation of *integration* in the word *integrity* encourages us to consider how we reconcile competing values and goods and how much we need practical wisdom to navigate the tensions that mark the moral landscape. Given the substantial overlap between the concepts of conscience and integrity, it is reasonable to treat them as largely interchangeable labels for a single moral domain.

Integrity takes on urgent meaning when utilitarian or other types of consequentialist reasoning motivate social arrangements or cooperative activities that focus so heavily on consequences that the value of individual moral action is discounted. Williams's notion of *moral projects* cuts against

[101] Childress, "Appeals to conscience."

the grain of utilitarianism, as it denies that the actions of an individual can be aggregated with the actions of other individuals into a single causal stream. For Williams, each person is deeply identified with, and morally responsible for, his or her own intentions and actions, which means that we should not treat an individual as if she were merely a channel for some larger causal stream that aggregates the sum total of everyone's interests and satisfactions. Final outcomes are not all that matters; how one gets to an outcome and who contributes to it are also morally relevant. The importance of individual moral responsibility is vital for understanding the significance of conscientious objection in medicine, in which the preservation of individual integrity can be seen as an irreducible value rather than merely one interest among many others.

Given the deep harmonies between conscience, unity, and moral integration, it may come as a surprise that some persons believe that an individual's conscience or integrity can be divided – we might say dis-integrated – into personal and professional domains. The question about the indivisible or divisible status of conscience or integrity has very practical implications for policy and law and for how we are to understand the moral origins of the beliefs and values that sustain the ethics, professionalism, and humanism that motivate and guide the practices of medical professionals. Those who treat conscience or integrity as divisible typically drive a wedge between the dichotomies of personal–professional, personal–public, or individual–professional, sometimes referring to "professional conscience" versus "individual conscience" or "personal integrity" versus "clinician integrity." Such partitioning is consistent with Walzer's view that both the self and its conscience are intrinsically divided by a multiplicity of internal moral voices.

But those who see moral agency or personhood as a unified whole believe that conscience and integrity are indivisible, and their rejection of divisibility addresses the problem that MacIntyre calls compartmentalization. A compartmentalized self lacks integrity because it is divided by different standards that change according to context or role. This kind of division can lead to moral distress when professionals feel forced to separate their individual and occupational values. The implausibility of drawing divisions through conscience or integrity is supported by Taylor's understanding of the inseparability of selfhood and moral meaning and the inescapability of moral frameworks. These frameworks allow us to find our place and orientation in the moral landscape, and they are defined by certain hypergoods – those goods we pursue that are incomparably higher than, or incommensurable with, other goods – which may include justice, benevolence, universal and equal respect for all persons, and the love of God. These hypergoods form the background against which we measure the worth of our lives and our endeavors.

In contrast to Walzer, Taylor and MacIntyre portray personal identity as unified by an orienting moral framework and an ongoing moral narrative. From this perspective, integrity is determined by an individual's life story as he encounters choices as opportunities that define his life by criteria and realities external to those choices. It is an integrity that does not merely ask, "What shall I do?" but also asks, "Who shall I be, and who shall I become?" If integrity is to reflect the moral need of physicians and other health care professionals to be complete and whole as persons, integrity requires the kind of vision that Taylor and MacIntyre are trying to encourage.

7

The Challenge and Inescapability of Moral Pluralism

Throughout the preceding chapters, I have discussed how moral beliefs and values play fundamental roles in clinical decision making and how we understand goals of care, practical wisdom, clinical judgment, conscience, and integrity. Whether taken for granted or explicitly stated, these beliefs and values reflect the assumptions and reasoning that guide the practice of medicine. I have also noted that in a morally pluralistic society, these beliefs and values will differ among individuals, and such differences will influence how patients and professionals make clinical decisions together and how political processes craft health policies.

Whether the differences arising from moral pluralism are expressed in philosophical or religious terms, they should be expected to be deeply rooted and broadly influential. Discussions related to such matters may at times take on a religious cast, since for many persons questions of morality or conscience are tied to moral foundations anchored in religious convictions. But of course this need not be so. Those who do not espouse religious beliefs still have deeply seated convictions that serve the same foundational role. Whether their convictions are described as philosophical or religious, all persons have what can be called *foundational beliefs* – that is, beliefs that serve as starting points for moral reasoning.

The challenges of moral pluralism are of central concern in this book. This chapter considers some of the implications of these challenges for medicine and ethics, in response to which I will recommend an inclusive understanding of foundational beliefs. According to this inclusive understanding, there is no ethically significant difference between a foundational belief that is labeled *religious* and one that is labeled *philosophical*. The basis for this inclusive approach arises from an appreciation of the similar foundational work these differently labeled beliefs perform in ethics, which is to define what people believe is *ultimately real* and *ultimately good.* Driving this discussion is the conviction that everyone who thinks about medicine and ethics must do so from one moral perspective or another, because there is no vantage point that is neutral or value-free. Each moral perspective entails foundational beliefs that reflect ultimate concerns. By way of illustration, consider how differently a sampling of persons may view a blastocyst. One person's beliefs about what is ultimately real and good lead to the conclusion that a blastocyst is human tissue that can legitimately be used as a source of human embryonic stem cells, and then discarded, in order to advance the cause of human health. Another person's beliefs about what is ultimately real and good lead to the conclusion that a blastocyst is an extremely early form of a human being and should not be sacrificed for others' purposes, no matter how noble those purposes may be. Our ethics depend on our beliefs.

I. MORAL PLURALISM AND RELIGIOUS BELIEF

There is a broad consensus in Western societies about the importance of a shared commitment to the values, structures, and procedures of constitutional democracy. There is also moral diversity in our societies that can test the extent and character of this shared commitment – as seen when strenuous debates arise over contentious questions of public policy and law. The source of this diversity arises from the foundational beliefs and values by which we assess the moral legitimacy of social practices and political arrangements. We can call the sum total of a person's foundational beliefs and values that person's moral framework, and it is through such frameworks that people perceive and engage their social environments in a moral way. Because of moral diversity, a multiplicity of moral frameworks pervades Western societies, creating the challenging reality of moral (or ethical) pluralism.

The existence of this pluralism is a focal point for those who note the contemporary absence of a socially shared moral framework and are concerned about its consequences. Jonathan Lear believes that we are morally at a loss because as a society we lack a coherent and compelling morality. We struggle, he says, to explain why we hold the moral beliefs we do, and we lack confidence in religion's ability to ground morality, which the Judeo-Christian tradition previously did in the West.[1] Jonathan Glover writes similarly, tracing the source of this loss back to a Nietzschean skepticism about a religious basis for morality (or any other metaphysical

[1] Lear, *Aristotle: the desire to understand*, 152.

or scientific basis, for that matter)[2] and suggesting that the prospects for reviving a shared belief in an objective moral law are dim.[3]

Though the practice of medicine enjoys a substantial degree of consensus about its primary purposes related to health and healing, the challenges of moral pluralism are still very real for the medical profession. Robert Veatch detects evidence of these challenges in the diverse content of medical codes and oaths, as well as the diversity of belief frameworks that surround, permeate, and influence the way clinicians practice.[4] Veatch sees potential for serious conflict between professionally generated norms and the religious and secular philosophical traditions in which physicians as individuals see themselves standing. He believes that in the face of such conflicts, we should expect physicians to give priority to their deeper (more foundational) commitments, which he presumes will be those based on their personal beliefs, whether religious or philosophical.

Pellegrino addresses the problem of moral diversity in medicine as it manifests in the variability of commitment to professional ideals among physicians. He sees a divide between physicians who avow the altruistic imperatives of medicine and those who do not. He recommends that we abandon the "illusion that all physicians share a common devotion to a high-flown set of ethical principles" and instead recognize the moral differences among physicians in such a way that allows patients "to choose among physicians on the basis of their ethical commitments as well as their reputations for technical expertise."[5] Pellegrino is candid not only about differences in values pertaining to professional ideals, but also about the religious diversity of physicians and the implications of their religious commitments for professional practice:

> For Catholics, Orthodox Jews, and Moslems, the teachings of the Gospel, Torah, or Koran take precedence in their lives and indeed inspire their healing vocations. For these major religions, healing the sick is ultimately a religious act and it comes ultimately from God. To practice medicine that contravenes religious teaching would be to subvert conscience to secular society and its "values," to act hypocritically, and to violate moral integrity intolerably.[6]

[2] Glover, *Humanity*, 11.
[3] Ibid., 41.
[4] Robert M. Veatch, "The sources of professional ethics: why professions fail," *Lancet* 373 (2009): 1000–1001.
[5] Pellegrino, "The virtuous physician, and the ethics of medicine," 252–53.
[6] Pellegrino, "The physician's conscience, conscience clauses, and religious belief."

Empirical observations suggest that religious beliefs among physicians are prevalent and influential. A study of 1,144 U.S. physicians revealed that 76 percent believe in God, 58 percent try hard to carry their religious beliefs over into all of their other dealings in life, and 55 percent report that their religious beliefs influence their practice of medicine.[7] Such findings suggest that assessments about the practice of medicine in a religiously and philosophically diverse society deserve the attention they receive by authors like Veatch and Pellegrino.

II. ABSENCE OF A NEUTRAL PERSPECTIVE

If philosophical and religious pluralism deprives the medical profession of a comprehensive moral consensus on foundational beliefs and values, it may be suggested that what medical practitioners need is a morally neutral stance that allows them to navigate the moral landscape of medical practice without advocating one particular moral framework over another. Some writers appear to believe this is possible, even necessary, when morally contentious issues are involved. For example, one finds suggestions that health care professionals should be "neutral arbiters of medical care,"[8] that they should provide "nondirective counseling" in which they refrain from "making, suggesting, or implying a recommendation,"[9] or that values and conscience (important parts of our private lives though they are) "should not influence the care an individual doctor offers to his or her patient."[10]

Such remarks suggest that it is possible for a health care professional to speak from a vantage point that is morally neutral or somehow detached from her own moral framework. I take such suggestions to be mistaken, because a morally detached or value-neutral vantage point is not available to morally attached practitioners in a value-loaded practice. Dan Brock stresses this point when he writes that it is not adequate to understand physicians "as value-neutral providers of the facts," since the reason physicians provide facts, and care, is always to promote a very basic value – the value of their patients' health.[11] Because health is considered a value, it is

[7] Farr A. Curlin et al., "Religious characteristics of U.S. physicians: a national survey," *Journal of General Internal Medicine* 20 (2005): 629–34.

[8] Cantor, "Conscientious objection gone awry."

[9] Chervenak and McCullough, "An ethically justified practical approach to offering, recommending, performing, and referring for induced abortion and feticide."

[10] Savulescu, "Conscientious objection in medicine."

[11] Brock, "Facts and values in the physician–patient relationship," 128.

a proper subject of our moral beliefs and values. The same is true for the goals of care deemed appropriate for health care. Writers who recognize the value-loaded nature of medical practice acknowledge that moral perspective and moral practice are inextricably linked. In the context of abortion, for instance, Dooley describes how claims of conscience derive from fundamental beliefs – be they religious, cultural, feminist, or political – and contrasting assessments of what is right and wrong arise from fundamentally different moral perspectives about the values at stake regarding women, the unborn, and society. "No morally neutral and non-question begging position can be found from which to judge conscientious refusals in abortion," she writes.[12] For Hauerwas, there is no neutral perspective, because all moral discernment depends on an understanding of the goods that form the end points of moral reasoning, goods that individuals come to recognize through the influence of their communities and traditions.[13] For Taylor, the diversity among these goods creates differences among persons which result in contrasting moral frameworks that simply do not allow for the possibility of a morally neutral vantage point.[14]

III. FRAGMENTATION OF MORAL VALUE AND THE DIVERSITY OF GOODS

As discussed thus far, the problem of moral pluralism arises from differences among persons that are normative (dealing with questions of right and wrong, good and bad) or metaethical (dealing with questions of meaning and justification).[15] This interpersonal pluralism is of considerable consequence for the practice of medicine and ethics. But there is another sense in which pluralism may be said to exist, and that is because of an irreconcilable plurality of values within ethics itself. On such a view, the ethical landscape itself is "plural" and therefore marked by fragmentation, not unity. It is important to keep this possible view in mind to avoid confusing interpersonal moral diversity with what some people believe is the intractably divided nature of ethical value itself.

Thomas Nagel is a prominent proponent of the view that moral value is fundamentally fragmented, and he underscores the challenge of

[12] Dolores Dooley, "Conscientious refusal to assist with abortion," *British Medical Journal* 309 (1994): 622–23.

[13] Hauerwas, "Reconciling the practice of reason," 139.

[14] Taylor, "The diversity of goods," 141.

[15] Frankena, *Ethics,* 11.

navigating one's way through a plurality of epistemic sources and contrasting normative values. He lays particular emphasis on the contrast between "the fragmentation of value and the singleness of decision,"[16] noting that, in the moral life, we are faced with any number of conflicting and incommensurable claims. Nevertheless, our practical moral circumstances require that amid these competing claims we act in a singular fashion by choosing one course of action over all others. Moral value is plural, he says, but moral decisions are singular. As a result there is a tension intrinsic to the moral life that defies resolution, and it can be traced to six basic types of moral value: specific obligations, rights, utility, perfectionist ends, private commitments, and self-interest. It is not possible to rank these values beside each other because they are irreducibly distinct. The root of the problem is anthropological, argues Nagel, because humans "are complex creatures who can view the world from many perspectives – individual, relational, impersonal, ideal, etc. – and each perspective presents a different set of claims."[17] Nagel believes it is a mistake to look for a unifying moral framework to resolve the dilemmas posed by the plurality of values, and he believes that looking "for a single general theory of how to decide the right thing to do is like looking for single theory of how to decide what to believe."[18]

Charles Taylor also offers an assessment of the contrasts between different kinds of moral value, an assessment that recognizes diverse goods in human life that form the basis of qualitative differences by which one can discriminate between different actions, feelings, and ways of living.[19] To illustrate his position, he describes the qualitative differences between integrity, charity, liberation, and rationality – differences that reveal the incommensurability of contrasts in the moral life and raise doubts as to how one can reconcile apparently incompatible values. Taylor criticizes the distorting attempt by utilitarianism or types of formalism (e.g., respect for moral personality) to eliminate the burden of this incompatibility by reducing the moral field to a single dimension. The moral life, he contends, does not lend itself to such reductionism, since the qualitative contrasts in our lives result in some modes of life, activities, and feelings being thought of as incommensurably higher than others.

[16] Nagel, "The fragmentation of value," 279.
[17] Ibid., 286.
[18] Ibid., 288.
[19] Taylor, "The diversity of goods."

Taylor would have us see that the moral life is not guided by a single overarching value, and he suggests that at least three kinds of moral valuation are relevant: the notion of utility (that which produces happiness is preferable to its opposite); the universal attribution of moral personality; and the variety of goals or virtues expressed in languages of qualitative contrast.[20] Though deep tensions run between these three kinds of valuation, Taylor holds that the task of the moral life includes the responsibility of prioritizing them throughout the course of a single life. Unlike Nagel's final assessment, Taylor believes that reconciliation among our highest moral commitments – which he calls hypergoods – is possible.[21] The possibility of such reconciliation points to the need for a unifying framework in the moral life, and this need brings us back to the question of foundational beliefs and, more specifically, to a consideration of those foundational beliefs that may be referred to as "religious."

IV. A MORE INCLUSIVE MEANING OF RELIGIOUS ETHICS BASED ON FOUNDATIONAL BELIEFS

Given the diverse meanings that can be attributed to religion and religious belief in a pluralistic society, we should clarify what *religion or theology* (as opposed to philosophy) and *religious or theological beliefs* (as opposed to philosophical beliefs) should be taken to signify in a discussion of ethics. According to standard accounts, religion entails beliefs, practices, communities, and a concept of God or notion of the Transcendent that can be described in terms of doctrine, sacred narrative, ritual, social institutions, experience, and ethics.[22] Laurence O'Connell and Martin Marty offer a functional explanation of religion that emphasizes its role in "addressing the existential, cognitive problem of meaning and the emotional, practical problem of adjusting to the material limits and frustrations inherent in individual human life and society," as well as its ability to provide "a plausible vision of the world and a viable means for getting around in it."[23] According to Courtney Campbell, religion "offers an interpretation or

[20] Ibid., 141.

[21] Taylor, *Sources of the self*, 107.

[22] Ninian Smart, "Religion," in *The Westminster dictionary of Christian theology*, ed. Alan Richardson and John Bowden (Philadelphia: Westminster Press, 1983), 496–98.

[23] Laurence J. O'Connell and Martin E. Marty, "Religious beliefs and bioethics: a crossed relationship," in *Notes from a narrow ridge: religion and bioethics*, ed. Dena S. Davis and Laurie Zoloth (Hagerstown, MD: University Publishing Group, 1999), 219.

revelation of reality that responds to what Max Weber referred to as the 'metaphysical needs of the human mind' to seek order, coherence, and meaning in our lives, to understand ultimate questions about our nature, purpose, and destiny."[24] The paramount importance of religious belief is captured succinctly by Paul Tillich's description of faith as a matter of "ultimate concern," demanding total commitment and promising ultimate fulfillment.[25]

On the basis of their relationship to universal human needs, some religious beliefs are relevant to all persons, whether or not those persons avow beliefs that they themselves would call religious. Such beliefs address universal needs for emotional support, cognitive satisfaction, and spiritual fulfillment that derive from basic human desires for meaning, purpose, hope, reconciliation, comfort, and courage. They concern questions about the value of human life, health, and embodiment; the value of human freedom; the meaning of disease, suffering, and death; the challenges of fallibility and finitude and the risk of overvaluing nonultimate things; and the value of serving and sacrificing for those who are weakened by illness and disability. Other areas addressed by religious beliefs usually entail an explicit belief in a transcendent being, whether or not that being is referred to as God. These areas include the role of gratitude (especially to a creator); the contrast between immanent and transcendent realities; the expectation of life after death; and the practical implications of believing in a personal God or some other omnipotent being to whom one gives one's deepest love or allegiance. The kinds of religious beliefs mentioned in this paragraph relate to the practice of medicine and ethics because they involve beliefs, needs, desires, or fears that apply directly to challenges posed by illness, suffering, disability, dependence, dying, and death.

For the purposes of this chapter, it is important to appreciate that religious beliefs do not only address existential or metaphysical concerns. Religious beliefs also perform essential ethical work in establishing the content of moral frameworks, because they provide foundational beliefs that serve as starting points for moral reasoning. And it is for this reason, in the context of ethics, that it is inappropriate to draw a line between one set of beliefs labeled *religious* and another set labeled *philosophical*,

[24] Courtney S. Campbell, "Religion and moral meaning in bioethics," *Hastings Center Report* 20, no. 4 (1990): S5.

[25] Paul Tillich, *Dynamics of faith* (New York: Harper & Row, 1957), 1–4.

because in doing so one fails to appreciate that beliefs under either of these labels serve similarly foundational roles in ethical reasoning.

This is the essential point John Reeder makes in an essay entitled "What Is a Religious Ethic?"[26] He argues that the stereotypical division between religious and nonreligious moral traditions in ethics is unwarranted if we expand our understanding of *religious* to include moral perspectives generally speaking, on the basis of the ethical significance of all fundamental beliefs and commitments regardless of whether they are called religious or nonreligious.[27] Reeder's thesis is that religions "search for the good in light of the limits and possibilities of the real" and that all moral traditions entail adopting one or another vision of what is good and real.[28] A vision of the *good* need not be extensive or complete, so long as it ranks some things over others. A vision of the *real* is necessary because our beliefs about reality will set the boundaries of our search for the good. The heuristic force of his inclusive categorization of "religious" is evident in the following summary:

> I have tried to sketch a concept of religion that emphasizes some aspects of what traditions have in common. Moreover, this concept, which insists that religions utilize *some* concept of the real in the search for the good, is intended to show how people who are often said to be nonreligious or secular should instead be said to have an alternative religion.... My basic point, then, is this: A tendency to define religion substantively in terms of a concern with an ontologically distinct reality (transcendent or immanent) or a nonconceivable mode of being can obscure the very important sense in which those who claim to have no religion are deeply religious.... the followers of Freud and Camus should see that they, too, attempt to "find their lives" through a vision of the real.[29]

[26] John P. Reeder, "What is a religious ethic?" *Journal of Religious Ethics* 25, no. 3 (suppl. S) (1998): 157–81.

[27] Reeder traces this inclusive view of religion to the work of Clifford Geertz. "If we adopt a concept of religion similar to Clifford Geertz's – which does not tie religion to a notion of God or even to a distinct sacred reality or object over against the profane, but locates its function as an orientation to the ultimately real, to basic elements and causes that influence human life for weal or woe – then we can say that both theological and philosophical ethics can be religious" (Clifford Geertz, "Religion as a cultural system," in *The interpretation of cultures* [New York: Basic Books, 1973], 87–125). John P. Reeder, "The dependence of ethics," in *James M. Gustafson's theocentric ethics: interpretations and assessments*, ed. Harlan R. Beckley and Charles M. Swezey (Macon, GA: Mercer University Press, 1988), 119–41.

[28] Reeder, "What is a religious ethic?" 160.

[29] Ibid., 167.

I accept Reeder's assessment and his conclusion that there is no convincing basis for a meaningful distinction between philosophical ethics and religious ethics[30] and that religious beliefs, in Reeder's inclusive sense, go all the way down to our moral foundations, reflecting what we take to be supremely important and fundamentally real. These are the foundations that "inevitably shape *all* moral convictions."[31]

When reading Reeder, it is important to keep in mind the contrast between things we might label, with a capital *R*, *Religious* (pertaining to beliefs about God and religious traditions, rituals, practices, communities, or institutions) and those things that occupy Reeder's attention and that we might label, with a small *r*, *religious* (pertaining to beliefs about what is real and good that ground our moral reasoning and reflect our ultimate concerns). In an effort to avoid potential misunderstandings and emphasize the shared significance of religious and philosophical beliefs when they play similarly foundational roles in moral reasoning, I prefer to use *foundational beliefs* to refer to these "small *r*" religious beliefs.

I believe that Reeder's analysis is highly instructive for medical ethics, and I rely on it in two ways. First, I accept that all moral frameworks in ethics function as religious ones do, because all frameworks make or imply claims about what is taken to be *ultimately real* and *ultimately good.* Second, I accept that each person's moral framework has particular implications, because the nature of a religious ethic – that is, the nature of foundational beliefs – is to go all the way down to the roots that supply the resources of a moral vision and nourish its practical manifestations.

V. THE UNAVOIDABILITY OF FOUNDATIONAL BELIEFS AND THEIR INFLUENCE ON MORAL FRAMEWORKS

Another way of expressing Reeder's assessment that all moral frameworks are religious is to say that foundational beliefs are unavoidable in the moral life. As Paul Ramsey put it, "everyone has an ultimate and no one leaves behind his unargued viewpoints when entering a rational argument."[32] Jeffrey Stout speaks of how indebted we are to our individual moral beginnings, since we do not start from scratch as morally reasoning persons but "begin already immersed in the assumptions and precedents

[30] Ibid., 175.

[31] Ibid., 171.

[32] Paul Ramsey, *Ethics at the edges of life* (Eugene, OR: Wipf & Stock, 2000), xv.

of a tradition, whether religious or secular," such that our starting points are "not so much arbitrary as inescapable."[33] Not only do all of us speak from our own moral vantage points, we also speak, notes Taylor, "from a moral orientation which we take to be right," an orientation that cannot simply be put on or taken off.[34]

In passing, it may be helpful to juxtapose the unavoidability of foundational beliefs to notions of impartiality, some discussions of which may suggest the need to surmount obstacles posed by one's personal standpoint.[35] Without meaning to deny the great value of impartiality in ethics, we should note that some descriptions of impartiality may risk creating expectations of attaining a moral vantage point that is somehow detached from the particular beliefs that define our moral lives – beliefs that might even be crucial in motivating a commitment to impartiality. If they are to reflect the unavoidable role of foundational beliefs, discussions of impartiality ought to take into account the way in which many people depend on frameworks of belief within their personal standpoints to decide moral issues. Kent Greenawalt expresses an appreciation for this in a discussion of religious beliefs, maintaining that it is neither plausible nor respectful to suggest that persons are supposed to approach moral reasoning by detaching themselves from their individual frameworks: "To demand that many devout Catholics, Protestants, and Jews pluck out their religious convictions is to ask them how they would think about a critical moral problem if they started from scratch, disregarding what they presently take as basic premises of moral thought."[36] The same objection would apply to nonreligious moral frameworks. We all have our own moral starting points, and we cannot detach ourselves from them. Our foundational beliefs are simply unavoidable.

[33] Jeffrey Stout, *Ethics after Babel: the languages of morals and their discontents* (Princeton, NJ: Princeton University Press, 2001), 120.

[34] Taylor, *Sources of the self*, 99.

[35] "Ethics always has to do with the conflict between the personal standpoint of the individual and some requirement of impartiality. The personal standpoint will bring in motives derived not only from the individual's interests but also from his attachments and commitments to people, projects, and particular things. The requirement of impartiality can take various forms, but it usually involves treating or counting everyone equally in some respect.... Since personal motives and impartiality can conflict, an ethical theory has to say something about how such conflicts are to be resolved." Thomas Nagel, "Moral conflict and political legitimacy," *Philosophy and Public Affairs* 16, no. 3 (1987): 215.

[36] Kent Greenawalt, *Religious convictions and political choice* (New York: Oxford University Press, 1988), 155.

VI. SUMMARY

Moral diversity in Western societies may at times test the consensus that democracies rely on to maintain shared commitments to policies and laws. This diversity stems from differences in the foundational beliefs and associated values that constitute the moral frameworks that allow individuals to understand themselves, their decisions, and the world in which they live. The diversity of moral frameworks creates the challenge of moral pluralism. Though the practice of medicine enjoys a substantial degree of moral consensus organized around its pursuit of health, the challenges of pluralism are nevertheless real for medical professionals, given the impact that diverse beliefs and values may have on understandings of health and on the goals of care that are deemed appropriate to promote and protect health. We cannot avoid the practical implications of pluralism by attempting to detach ourselves from our moral frameworks or achieve a morally neutral position. Each person speaks from some moral vantage point, and a value-neutral position is not available in a practice like medicine that is inherently value-loaded.

There is also a sense in which moral pluralism arises from ethics itself, because of the multiple competing values that make up the moral realm and give rise to many dilemmas – values such as obligations to others, rights, utility, private commitments, and self-interest. Ethical decision making can be vexing because it demands a single course of action amid a multiplicity of competing values or because it requires prioritizing multiple values. The apparent incommensurability of fundamental moral values (hypergoods) raises the question of prioritization in the moral life and the need for a guiding orientation provided by a framework of moral value. This need cannot be addressed without engaging questions about our deepest beliefs, which requires consideration of beliefs commonly referred to as "religious."

Given the role religious beliefs play in moral pluralism, it is important to clarify what *religious*, as opposed to *philosophical*, beliefs signify in the context of ethics. For this purpose, it is important to keep in mind the contrast between things we might label *Religious* (with a capital *R*) – pertaining to beliefs about God, as well as religious traditions, rituals, practices, communities, and institutions – and things we might label *religious* (with a small *r*) – pertaining to beliefs about what is real and good – that play fundamental roles in our moral reasoning. I call the latter beliefs *foundational beliefs* to indicate the commonality between religious and philosophical beliefs when they play similarly basic roles in moral reasoning. This commonality marks the inclusive character of foundational beliefs and explains why the stereotypical division between religious and nonreligious moral traditions in ethics can be set aside once we recognize that *all* moral frameworks make claims about what we believe is ultimately good and what we recognize as ultimately real. Because all moral frameworks make such claims, foundational beliefs are unavoidable in moral reasoning. These foundational beliefs form the basis of our moral frameworks, and they inevitably have practical manifestations.

Foundational beliefs represent the moral background of ethical deliberation. We all rely on foundational beliefs for our moral starting points – whether explicitly defined or casually assumed – and we should not pretend to be able to manage without them. Acknowledgment of these beliefs may be minimal or absent when ethics is discussed in terms of virtues, principles, or consequences. And even when people acknowledge the challenges of interpreting, balancing, and integrating such sources of ethical value, there may still be silence regarding the guiding role that foundational beliefs play in moral reasoning. If ethical deliberation in medicine is to do justice to our moral frameworks, it must be ready to recognize and engage the foundational beliefs that guide our judgments and shape our decisions.

8

Implications of Moral Pluralism for Public Dialogue and Professional Practice

The preceding chapter discussed the challenge of moral pluralism, a challenge that cannot be met by supposing there can be a morally neutral vantage point from which to address ethically challenging aspects of medical practice. Pluralism exists not only among persons but also within ethics itself, due to contrasts between different basic moral goods. The chapter addressed the need for an inclusive understanding of foundational beliefs – one that relates to all persons regardless of their religious or philosophical affiliations, since everyone works within a moral framework based on assumptions about what is ultimately real and ultimately good. These foundational beliefs serve as starting points for moral reasoning, and they are as unavoidable as they are vital.

If ethical decision making in medicine ought to encourage integrity among physicians through the integration of their beliefs, values, and actions, then foundational beliefs have to be acknowledged and their significance respected. But in a morally pluralistic setting, questions arise about the extent to which professionals should be allowed to refer to, and act on, their foundational beliefs in their professional practice. These kinds of questions have led to strenuous debates beyond the medical context (i.e., in society at large), especially when foundational beliefs are labeled "religious" and the setting is the "public square" of civic activity or political deliberation. Some people oppose the idea of citizens referring to reasons based on religious beliefs to promote public policies or social practices when those reasons are thought to be incomprehensible to citizens who do not share them. Others counter by maintaining that such opposition is unfounded, since there is no compelling distinction between reasons considered "religious" (putatively accessible only to some) and reasons considered "public" (and putatively accessible to all).

In the midst of moral pluralism and debates about the kinds of reasons that should be allowed in public life, how should medical professionals engage in moral dialogues (with each other, with patients, and with society), and what kinds of reasons should they be allowed to offer as they pursue what they believe is the ethical practice of medicine? This chapter focuses on these and other questions regarding where moral pluralism leaves the medical professional with respect to public dialogue and professional practice.

I. OPPOSITION TO REFERENCES TO RELIGIOUS BELIEFS IN PUBLIC LIFE

Observers of the way in which religious beliefs are treated in bioethical discourse have voiced concern that religious language and narrative are not welcome in secular debates about medical practice or health care policy. Lisa Cahill sees such opposition arising from the demand that bioethical arguments be open to rational scrutiny or else excluded from public discussion, a demand based on the belief that religious convictions represent a form of fanaticism that is disruptive to public moral dialogues.[1] Courtney Campbell believes that the academic bioethics community functions on the assumption that religious beliefs are largely irrelevant to ethics, suggesting that in public contexts, scholars who work within religious traditions are forced to convey their contributions in terms that can be understood by those outside their religious communities, thereby restricting discussion to the domain of nonreligious moral categories.[2] The result of such concessions, claims Basil Mitchell, is a contracted view that excludes religion by cutting off argument at the point where people's deeper convictions become decisively relevant.[3] Assuming such concerns have at least some validity, it may be possible to shed some light on their sources by considering how references to religious beliefs are treated more generally in discussions about public policy and law.

Among political philosophers, there are some who insist that public deliberative processes in a liberal democracy appropriately exclude

[1] Lisa Sowle Cahill, "Theology and bioethics: should religious traditions have a public voice?" *Journal of Medicine and Philosophy* 17 (1992): 265.

[2] Courtney S. Campbell, "Bearing witness: religious resistance and meaning," in *Notes from a narrow ridge: religion and bioethics*, ed. Dena S. Davis and Laurie Zoloth (Hagerstown, MD: University Publishing Group, 1999), 24, 41–42.

[3] Basil Mitchell, "The role of theology in bioethics," in *Theology and bioethics*, ed. E. E. Shelp (Dordrecht: Reidel, 1985), 77.

religious beliefs and values from public discussions and debates about political and legal decisions. They typically base their positions on the claim that religious beliefs and values do not satisfy the demands of "public reason," which, it is said, supplies justification for state-sanctioned actions and policies in terms that are accessible (i.e., understandable) to reasonable persons. This demand for accessibility arises from the recognition that political power is coercive and from the belief that such coercion is tolerable only when it can be justified in terms accessible to those who are coerced. Insisting on such a constraint, it is argued, honors the autonomy of persons who must abide by laws that restrict their liberty. The putative impropriety of making reference to religious beliefs in public moral debates therefore assumes there is a tenable distinction between reason-based and faith-based beliefs that separates moral reasons that are public and accessible (and therefore relevant) from religious reasons that are private and inaccessible (and therefore irrelevant).

John Rawls was an influential contributor to the debate over the role of religious belief in the public square.[4] In *A Theory of Justice* (1971) he proposed a moral justification for a conception of right and justice within the tradition of Enlightenment liberalism,[5] and this justification was not supposed to depend on any comprehensive moral frameworks. In *Political Liberalism* (1993), however, he acknowledged that Enlightenment liberalism is as comprehensive a framework as any religious doctrine. He therefore abandoned hope for a full justification of a theory of justice, focusing instead on a partial justification limited to political (as opposed to metaphysical) values. In *Political Liberalism* he endeavored to find a basis for a reasonable common ground in the midst of reasonable pluralism.

The problem, as Rawls saw it, is that modern democratic society is characterized by a pluralism of incompatible yet reasonable comprehensive doctrines (whether religious, political, or moral). This pluralism is the expected result of the exercise of human reason under free and enduring institutions. Rawls asked: How can such deeply opposed comprehensive doctrines coexist and support the political conception of a constitutional democracy? His answer was to work out a conception of political justice that a plurality of reasonable doctrines might endorse without replacing

4 In this discussion I assess Rawls's arguments related to his conception of public reason as he expressed them in *Political Liberalism* (1993), "Political Liberalism and Religion" (a paper presented at Yale in 1994), and *The Idea of Public Reason Revisited* (1997). These arguments are unchanged in Rawls's last published volume (John Rawls, *Justice as fairness: a restatement*, ed. Erin Kelly [Cambridge, MA: Harvard University Press, 2001]).

5 John Rawls, "Political liberalism and religion" (Yale University, October 6–7, 1994).

any comprehensive doctrines or establishing their foundations. Such a conception would be defined by an overlapping consensus that is independent of all comprehensive doctrines ("free-floating") but still sustained by the capacity of those comprehensive doctrines for deeper and fuller moral justification. Rawls believed that this consensus is not merely a modus vivendi; if it were only that, the consensus would be susceptible to the vicissitudes of contingent circumstances and would therefore be unreliable as the basis of a stable constitutional democracy.

Rawls's idea of an overlapping consensus is one that is expected to be acknowledged by all citizens according to the dictates of human reason, as formalized in the liberal principle of legitimacy, which holds that "our exercise of political power is fully proper only when it is exercised in accordance with a constitution the essentials of which all citizens as free and equal may reasonably be expected to endorse in the light of principles and ideals acceptable to their common human reason."[6] The liberal principle of legitimacy is closely tied to Rawls's idea of public reason, the content of which is independent of all comprehensive doctrines. This notion of public reason, which makes public justification possible, is the only legitimate form of reason when constitutional essentials and basic justice are at stake. For such fundamental concerns, "we are only to appeal to presently accepted general beliefs and forms of reasoning found in common sense, and the methods and conclusions of science when these are not controversial."[7] Public reason insists that citizens be able to explain even their votes to one another by reasons that are composed of public political values. Comprehensive doctrines that fail to offer such explanations cannot be considered "reasonable."

Rawls discusses the limits of public reason and considers when, if ever, reasons expressed in terms of comprehensive doctrines may legitimately enter public discourse. An "exclusive view" would entirely prohibit any reference to the doctrinal beliefs that support a public reason. An "inclusive view" would leave room, on occasion, for the presentation of the comprehensive basis of a political value, provided this was done "in ways that strengthen the ideal of public reason itself."[8] Rawls refers here to a comprehensive *basis*, not a comprehensive *reason*, since the reason given is always a public one. Rawls cites Martin Luther King and Abraham Lincoln

[6] John Rawls, *Political liberalism* (New York: Columbia University Press, 1993), 137.
[7] Ibid., 224.
[8] Ibid., 247.

as public figures who referred appropriately to their comprehensive doctrinal beliefs.

In "Political Liberalism and Religion" (1994) Rawls offered further definitions of "reasonable" and elaborated on the contrast between public reason and religious belief. This work states that one of the basic tenets of liberalism is a "stress on the social world's being explicable to the reason of every last individual,"[9] since only generally explicable reasons can justify political power, which is always coercive. The concern to justify the structures of political power in a constitutional democracy drives his search for the *idea* of a political conception of justice (the *content* of which would be filled in by the parties in the "original position"). In "Political Liberalism and Religion," Rawls's description of "reasonable" is that which expresses a reflective attitude to toleration and a form of conduct whereby citizens communicate their mutual respect for each other. His discussion in "Political Liberalism and Religion" also revisits the "exclusive" and "inclusive" views mentioned earlier and expresses preference for a "wide view," with an acknowledgment that in *Political Liberalism* he took too narrow a view of public reason. This more accommodating stance recognizes two instances in which reference to comprehensive doctrinal beliefs can be appropriate: (1) in highly contested political disputes (if doing so would actually foster the duty of civility) and (2) in an unjust society (so long as comprehensive beliefs support constitutional values). Rawls then makes what he considers a further concession, stating that citizens "may freely introduce their reasonable comprehensive doctrines, with one crucial proviso: namely, that in due course they support the political measures they propose in terms of the principles and values of the public political conception of justice."[10]

In *The Idea of Public Reason Revisited* (1997), Rawls repeated his core arguments and emphasized that on his account public reason "neither criticizes nor attacks any comprehensive doctrine, religious or nonreligious, except insofar as that doctrine is incompatible with the essentials of public reason and a democratic polity."[11] In public political dialogue, citizens should think of themselves as if they were legislators and exercise political power by giving reasons that would be acceptable if issued by government officials. Rawls acknowledges that those who rely on their

[9] Rawls, "Political liberalism and religion," 2.

[10] Ibid., 26–27.

[11] John Rawls, "The idea of public reason revisited," *University of Chicago Law Review* 64, no. 3 (1997): 766.

own comprehensive doctrines (religious or secular) for what they believe to be the truths relevant to political life will reject his idea of public reason. But he stresses his conviction that the conception of public reason he supports is *not* secular reason.

> We must distinguish public reason from what is sometimes referred to as secular reason or secular values. These are not the same as public reason. For I define secular reason as reasoning in terms of comprehensive nonreligious doctrines. Such doctrines and values are much too broad to serve the purposes of public reason. Political values are not moral doctrines, however available or accessible these may be to our reason and common sense reflection. Moral doctrines are on a level with religion and first philosophy. By contrast, liberal political principles and values, although intrinsically moral values, are specified by liberal political conceptions of justice and fall under the category of the political.[12]

In *The Idea of Public Reason Revisited* Rawls continued to maintain that the substance of our comprehensive doctrines may be introduced into political discussion, but only if in due course we also give proper public reasons for the principles and policies we support. He objected to any direct movement from a comprehensive doctrine to a political value that is not accompanied by an independent justification resting on his conception of public reason. For instance, anyone who would choose to make a political point by invoking the parable of the Good Samaritan could not begin and end with a story about a man on the road to Jericho. Any use of the parable would have to be followed by a public justification for the parable's conclusions in terms of political values.[13] For Rawls such stories are redundant elaborations, not independent justifications.

Rawls claimed to have put aside all accounts of human nature in his political conception of justice by proposing a political conception of persons as citizens. His argument would attempt to persuade us that on his view there need be no war between religion and democracy, since political liberalism rejects the Enlightenment liberalism that historically attacked Christianity. His only requirement for all the comprehensive doctrines that form a reasonable overlapping consensus is that each one must affirm the political institutions of a constitutional democratic society, that is, "equal basic rights and liberties for all citizens, including liberty of conscience and the freedom of religion."[14]

[12] Ibid., 775–76.
[13] Ibid., 786.
[14] Ibid., 801.

Like Rawls, Thomas Nagel opposes reference to religious reasons to justify public arguments because he believes that the grounds for any form of political coercion must be justifiable on terms acceptable to all citizens, not just those who share a particular set of beliefs. Accordingly, Nagel argues for an epistemic restraint that distinguishes between what is needed to justify one's individual beliefs and what is needed to justify the employment of political power. Political dialogue, he argues, takes us to our highest framework of moral reasoning, to a standpoint outside ourselves and independent of who we are. Liberal impartiality requires that the beliefs we use to justify our public policies be justifiable from an impersonal standpoint. For Nagel, this means that "we may have to regard certain of our beliefs, whether moral or religious or even historical or scientific, simply as someone's beliefs, rather than as truths – unless they can be given the kind of impersonal justification appropriate to [the political] perspective, in which case they may be appealed to as truths without qualification."[15] This moral impersonalization requires an epistemic division between the private and the public domains to distinguish between what are and are not acceptable grounds for the use of political power by the majority. Disagreements ought to be adjudicated not by assertions and counterassertions involving contrasting beliefs, but by submission to objective common ground. Nagel objects to religious beliefs in political dialogue because they fail to provide such common ground. Political justification requires

> that it must be possible to present to others the basis of your beliefs, so that once you have done so, *they have what you have,* and can arrive at a judgment on the same basis. That is not possible if part of the source of your conviction is personal faith or revelation – because to report your faith or revelation to someone else is not to give him what you have, as you do when you show him your evidence or give him your arguments.[16]

Robert Audi's portrayal of the place of religious beliefs in public discussion is similar to the descriptions by Rawls and Nagel and shares with their accounts a central concern with the justification of political coercion. Audi argues that liberal democracy resists coercion and prefers persuasion, because we tend to do autonomously that of which we ourselves are persuaded. When there must be coercion, liberal democracies attempt to justify it by reference to considerations that any rational adult

[15] Nagel, "Moral conflict and political legitimacy," 230.
[16] Ibid., 232.

citizen would find persuasive.[17] He offers the principles of secular rationale and secular motivation,[18] defining secular reason as reason that "does not evidentially depend on the existence of God (or denying it) or on theological considerations, or on the pronouncements of a person or institution *qua* religious authority."[19] He also puts forward what he calls the notion of "mixed obligational overdetermination," by which he allows for religious believers to inject their comprehensive views into public debate for justification and motivation, so long as sufficient secular reasons are also invoked. In this allowance Audi believes himself to stand in contrast to Rawls. But Rawls's adoption of the "wide view" in "Political Liberalism and Religion" appears very similar to Audi's. Moreover, in another way Audi's position offers less than Rawls's, with respect to the religious and secular varieties of comprehensive doctrines, for unlike Rawls, Audi singles out religious doctrines for criticism and leaves their secular counterparts alone.

In contrast to Rawls, William Galston argues that there can be no neutral description of liberal theory and that liberalism must be frank about *its* conception, however thin, of the human good. He insists that Rawls is incorrect to suppose that good social theory is political, not metaphysical.[20] Accompanying Galston's assessment of liberal theory and the good is a recognition that both sides in the culture wars of our generation need to moderate their most extreme claims. While he does not address the epistemic basis for his concept of rationality, he offers a definition for it that includes the requirement that, in public deliberation, citizens should have the disposition to employ public reasons that are open to inspection by others, whenever possible.[21] While the qualification "whenever possible" seems at first glance to make this requirement seem more an invitation than a demand, in his chapter on public virtue and religion Galston makes it clear that religious believers must realize which of their beliefs can, and which cannot, be introduced to public discussion.

[17] Robert Audi and Nicholas Wolterstorff, *Religion in the public square* (Lanham, MD: Rowman & Littlefield, 1997), 16.

[18] Ibid., 25, 28–29. The principle of secular rationale: "One has a prima facie obligation not to advocate or support any law or public policy that restricts human conduct, unless one has, and is willing to offer, adequate secular reason for this advocacy or support (say for one's vote)." The principle of secular motivation: "One has a (prima facie) obligation to abstain from advocacy or support of a law or public policy that restricts human conduct, unless one is sufficiently *motivated* by (normatively) adequate secular reason."

[19] Ibid., 26.

[20] William Galston, *Liberal purposes* (Cambridge: Cambridge University Press, 1991), 37.

[21] Ibid., 175–76.

"For their part, moral and religious traditionalists must learn to distinguish between the portion of their creed that can play a legitimate role in the public sphere and the portion that must remain within the confines of group practice or individual conscience."[22] While Galston is forthright in his depiction of liberalism as a theory of the good, his treatment of rationality and the role of religion (tradition) appears to assume a notion of public reason similar to that of Rawls, Nagel, and Audi – except that Galston is also prepared to accept traditional moral or religious values so long as they prove to be supportive of liberal politics or result in social policies that can be justified by consequentialist appeals. In contrast to Rawls and Audi, Galston does not require a form of justificatory overdetermination when appeals to religious beliefs are made.

II. SUPPORT FOR REFERENCES TO RELIGIOUS BELIEFS IN PUBLIC LIFE

The authors discussed in the preceding section believe that the proper function of democratic societies depends on notions of public reason that disqualify or limit religious beliefs when it comes to public discussions about policies and laws. But there are also philosophers who believe such restrictions on religious beliefs are unfounded and unfair. One of these is Nicholas Wolterstorff. To understand the issues at stake in this discussion, it is helpful to consider his assessment of the assumptions that underlie much of the debate. He is particularly concerned with the epistemological restraints that liberal theorists impose on religious believers to prohibit them from using religious reasons to determine their public arguments.[23] These restraints arise from a commitment to what is known as foundationalism, in which rational beliefs about life and the universe are either basic (part of the foundation) or nonbasic (supported by the foundation). As Alvin Plantinga describes, foundationalism requires that, for a belief to be basic, it has to be self-evident, incorrigible, or evident to the senses.[24] By contrast, nonbasic beliefs are traceable to, and therefore justified by, basic beliefs. What is important to appreciate here is the restriction foundationalism places on the kinds of beliefs that are allowed

22 Ibid., 257.
23 Audi and Wolterstorff, *Religion in the public square*, 69.
24 Alvin Plantinga, "Reason and belief in God," in *Faith and rationality: reason and belief in God*, ed. Alvin Plantinga and Nicholas Wolterstorff (Notre Dame, IN: University of Notre Dame Press, 1983), 16–93.

to stand on their own – that is, a restriction on what beliefs are allowed to be taken as foundational.

Wolterstorff and Plantinga are among philosophers of religion who have argued rigorously against foundationalism. They reject the assumption that because religious beliefs involving faith in God do not satisfy the restrictive requirements of foundationalism, such beliefs should not be allowed in the public square to support or oppose public policies. Against the assumptions of foundationalism, Wolterstorff asserts:

> Not only is it not the case that one must hold one's religious beliefs for reasons of the Lockean sort to be entitled to them, it is not, in general, necessary that one hold them for any reasons at all. Something about the belief, the person, and the situation brings it about that the person is entitled to the belief.[25]

Wolterstorff points out that the foundationalist critics of religious belief generally make an assumption about the existence of a common rationality that is supposed to supply criteria for determining which beliefs are foundational. Wolterstorff argues, however, that rationality in what we believe is not what these critics claim it is. Instead, he argues that we are endowed with belief dispositions that give rise to what are referred to as *immediate* beliefs. Some of these dispositions we share with most other human beings, some we do not. Thus conceived, rationality is contextual and situation-specific – that is, it is always *situated*. In contrast to those who insist that theistic convictions must be reinforced by more fundamental beliefs through a process of inference, Wolterstorff maintains that

> a person is rationally justified in believing a certain proposition which he does believe unless he has adequate reason to cease from believing it. Our beliefs are rational unless we have reason for refraining; they are not nonrational unless we have reason *for* believing. They are innocent until proved guilty, not guilty until proved innocent.[26]

Wolterstorff also points to a simple problem of logic related to the evidence requirements of foundationalism: "How, if we are going to trust no belief disposition whatsoever until proved reliable, are we going to prove it reliable?"[27] Some beliefs must be assumed to be reliable before the process of proving can begin. Wolterstorff maintains that we must always situate the question of the rationality of a belief – for instance, a

[25] Audi and Wolterstorff, *Religion in the public square*, 87.

[26] Nicholas Wolterstorff, "Can belief in God be rational if it has no foundations?" in *Faith and rationality*, ed. Plantinga and Wolterstorff, 163.

[27] Ibid., 174–75.

belief in God – in relation to a particular person in a particular context. The belief system of such a person must be scrutinized before the rationality of her religious beliefs can be judged.

Wolterstorff offers a multifaceted critique of Rawls's idea of public reason as found in *Political Liberalism.* First, he argues that Rawls is not justified in his assumption that the idea of liberal democracy can be retrieved from the shared political culture of certain extant societies. Rawls relies upon the *consensus populi* as the political basis of a constitutional democracy, but Wolterstorff believes he works with "an extraordinarily idealized picture of the American mind," as if gazing through the rose-tinted glasses of the idea of liberal democracy.[28] Second, Wolterstorff notes the exegetical industry it would require to understand what Rawls means by "reasonable" and "rational," and he expresses concern over what he perceives to be Rawls's lack of epistemic articulation. He argues that Rawls fails to inform us of the content of public reason and, more fundamentally, that he does not recognize that human reason is always "programmed" human reason. Third, the demand that all citizens adopt public reason does not take into account people's comprehensive particularities and prevents them from living fully integrated lives; this is unfair for those who are deeply committed to integrating their religious beliefs with their choices and actions.[29] Wolterstorff completes his criticism of Rawls by faulting him for trying to discover and develop a shared political basis for a communitarian politics that cannot be found and for failing to accept that we must learn to live with a politics that is composed of multiple communities.[30]

As already mentioned, the liberal political requirement that reasons used in public be generally accessible typically arises from the claim that coercive power can be justified only when the reasons for coercion are intelligible to those persons coerced so that disrespect for individual autonomy is avoided. This fundamental claim rests on two assumptions: (1) that there is such a thing as "public reason" and (2) that we dishonor each other when we support laws and political policies for reasons that are not shared by all those who will be affected by them. The first assumption is undermined, I believe, by Wolterstorff's argument that liberal political theorists typically fail to make their epistemology explicit and, even when they do make their dependence on evidentialism known (as in the case of

28 Audi and Wolterstorff, *Religion in the public square*, 97.
29 Ibid., 116.
30 Ibid., 109.

Locke), foundationalist claims prove mistaken: if all rationality is really *situated*, all reference to "public reason" is, strictly speaking, pretense. The second assumption, while perhaps plausible on its face, is not finally compelling in the setting of a liberal democracy. Why should disagreement be allowed over policies but not over the reasons for those policies? I think Wolterstorff is right to conclude that consensus in our reasons is neither foreseeable nor necessary as we carry on in our ad hoc political efforts to engineer the compromises that lead to policies and laws within a peaceable democracy.

Another contributor to the debate over the proper place of religious beliefs in public moral dialogues is Jürgen Habermas. In his 2005 Holberg Lecture, entitled "Religion in the Public Sphere," Habermas discusses what he calls the "asymmetrical burden" that the Rawlsian separation of religious and secular language imposes on people whose religious faith nurtures their entire lives. It is an imposition because for these people religious faith represents "a mode of believing that infuses the very pores of daily life," and the burden results in cognitive dissonance when they are compelled to act as if religious beliefs can be set aside in the public sphere.[31] Habermas argues that a society that requires an institutional separation of religion and politics must not transform that requirement into an "undue mental and psychological burden" for those citizens who have moral and political commitments deriving from religious faith. Such citizens must not, he maintains, be expected to "split their identity in public and private components" as they participate in public debates and contribute to the political process.

Habermas engages Wolterstorff's critique of Rawls's objection to religious references and justifications in public political discourse and in so doing acknowledges that the Rawlsian restriction should be loosened somewhat. Habermas bases his position on two claims. First, he believes that the liberal state has an interest in including religious voices in political debates in order to avoid depriving secular society of important religious insights regarding social forms of dignified human living that might otherwise be lost. He believes these insights may have a normative truth content that can be translated into generally accessible moral language and may prove useful in secular society, perhaps even capturing intuitions among nonreligious persons that have been obscured. Second, Habermas believes that moral and political dialogue in the public

[31] Jürgen Habermas, "Religion in the public sphere" (Jürgen Habermas and the Holberg Prize, 2005).

sphere places a bilateral burden on all those who participate, and in this dialogue religious citizens should not be encumbered with an asymmetrical burden of translation. He suggests that translation of religious insights into generally accessible language should be seen as a cooperative task and a shared responsibility. "Whereas citizens of faith may make public contributions in their own religious language only subject to the proviso that these get translated, the secular citizens must open their minds to the possible truth content of those presentations and even enter into dialogues from which religious reasons then might emerge in the transformed guise of generally accessible arguments."

Habermas's perspective is distinct in its move toward shared responsibility for dialogue and translation between secular and religious persons involved in political and moral dialogue, and to this extent he advances beyond the Rawlsian position. However, he still situates himself firmly within the Rawlsian framework by insisting that when political decisions are enforced by the state through the crafting of policy and law, their justifications must be formulated in language that is equally accessible to all citizens. It should be added that Habermas's central focus appears to be on restrictions regarding religious references that should apply to government leaders, in contrast to Rawls and others who would apply such restrictions not only to legislators, but also to citizens who speak in the public sphere. Like Rawls, Habermas favors prohibiting religious expression and justification among law and policy makers in the absence of a parallel justification expressed in secular terms. But unlike Rawls, he favors allowing religious expression by citizens in the public square and exhorts all parties, secular and religious, to engage in the shared work of dialogue and translation.

III. MEDICAL PROFESSIONALS: CITIZENS, PUBLIC OFFICIALS, OR SOMETHING IN BETWEEN?

For Rawls, Nagel, Wolterstorff, and Habermas, the focus of discussion is the political role of individuals as citizens, or that of elected officials as legislators, in a morally and religiously pluralistic democracy. How should this discussion bear on the practice of medicine and the responsibilities of medical professionals? Should we view medical professionals as we do elected officials, since both have socially sanctioned and supported roles that carry obligations to promote the public good? Or are medical professionals more like other (unelected) citizens, with more freedom to decide how to live their role-specific lives than can be expected of elected officials, who for good reasons are sometimes also called public servants? By virtue of the "social contract" between the medical profession and society, which will be discussed later, physicians clearly have social expectations attached to their roles. And the balance of freedom and obligation within these role expectations presumably lies somewhere between nonphysician citizens and elected officials. How much freedom and how much obligation are attributed to a physician's professional role will depend heavily on one's assessment of the expectations of the social contract.

With respect to the preceding discussion, we may note that the debate among political philosophers about the legitimacy of references to religious beliefs in public contexts focuses on public justifications for laws and policies, not the practices of individual medical professionals. The core issue for writers like Rawls and Nagel is the need to be able to explain the bases for government decisions, which are by nature coercive in their effect on the lives of citizens. In the "wide view" Rawls advocated in "Political Liberalism and Religion," he held that it may be acceptable to refer to comprehensive doctrinal beliefs (1) in highly contested political disputes (if doing so would actually foster the duty of civility) or (2) in an unjust society (so long as comprehensive beliefs support constitutional values).[32] In medicine, the first of these two conditions would appear to justify "wide" accommodations in highly contested practices such as abortion and physician-assisted suicide.

As for Nagel, his conception of liberal impartiality insists on a division between private and public domains that distinguishes between reasons that are and are not acceptable justifications for the use of political power by the majority. One wonders whether Nagel would favor the application of such a division to determine the kinds of reasons that are ethically acceptable in decision making shared by patients and physicians. Perhaps he would not place the same epistemic demands on individual physicians as he would on a political majority – unless he envisions patients as being as vulnerable to coercion by physicians as political minorities are to political majorities.

IV. PERSONAL SIGNIFICANCE OF MORAL DIALOGUE

The significance of the discussion in the first two sections of this chapter can be summarized as a concern about fairness with respect to the kinds of reasons (e.g., religious vs. nonreligious) that should be considered

[32] Rawls, "Political liberalism and religion," 26–27.

acceptable in the public square. But there is another reason some observers believe in the importance of ensuring that people are free to refer to their religious or other comprehensive beliefs in the course of their interpersonal moral dialogues generally speaking. This reason is articulated by Charles Taylor, and it arises from what is called the *dialogical* character of moral life. This communicative aspect of moral identity and formation invites us to see that we recognize and form our moral identities through our dialogues with other persons, not in individualistic isolation.[33] Our moral identities are sustained and cultivated through communication with others throughout our lives, and as a result we can be described as "dialogical selves." Taylor describes this dialogical reality as a web of interlocution through which we all exist as selves and come to understand our selves.[34] He also maintains that we have a need to articulate our moral sources and that the act of articulation "can bring us closer to the good as a moral source, can give it power."[35] For Taylor, expressing the beliefs and values that we love or respect is an act that communicates our commitments to others and also empowers us to be good.

Taylor's perspective helps us see how dialogue with patients and colleagues can help medical professionals engage the value-loaded landscape of medicine, especially when contrasting values are contested and lead to conflicts. Such dialogue can enhance a professional's self-understanding and strengthen his resolve to do his moral best. The act of articulating foundational beliefs and values in an effort to explain reasoning and decision making can thereby facilitate personal growth, as those beliefs and values are allowed to harmonize with words and actions. On Taylor's account, the act of moral communication therefore has a twofold significance: it is *informative*, in that it shows respect for patients and colleagues by providing reasons for morally significant actions, and it is *performative*, in that it nourishes a professional's integrity by reinforcing moral commitments and strengthening identity.

V. PROCEDURALISM: A LIMITED RESPONSE TO THE PREDICAMENT OF MORAL PLURALISM

Debates about the public acceptability of making reference to religious beliefs in discussions of policy or law reflect the degree to which

[33] Taylor, *The ethics of authenticity*, 33–35.
[34] Taylor, *Sources of the self*, 36.
[35] Ibid., 92.

moral pluralism pervades and potentially divides Western societies. In Wolterstorff's assessment, this pluralism goes so far as to encompass notions of rationality itself and imply that we must be content to live within the politics of multiple moral communities due to our lack of a broad moral consensus. In the context of bioethics, this absence of consensus led Basil Mitchell to suggest that moral diversity has forced us to dig at the roots of our contrasting moral intuitions and, as a result, acknowledge the existence of our profound and disturbing differences.[36] H. Tristram Engelhardt offers a sobering assessment of these differences and locates their origins in the demise of the shared moral fabric that once characterized Western societies. He argues that we are now in the ruins of a Christian heritage that holds mere "fragments of moral intuitions from a once intact way of life."[37] Moreover, we have also lost the Enlightenment's confidence in a rationally coherent and universally accessible moral narrative. Taken together, these result in a secular bioethics that is plural, marked by multiple moral visions and the implausibility of any claims to absolute truth. For Engelhardt, the deep pluralism of our contemporary context means that the secular bioethical community is rationally incapable of deciding between competing foundational premises.[38]

Engelhardt traces the origins of the predicament of our postmodern age to the moral and canonical fracture begun by the Reformation, after which the Western Christian moral narrative failed to hold, and secular morality could not make up the deficiency. "After the fragmentation of the Reformation and the secularization of the Enlightenment, there is the moral diversity of post-modernity."[39] Engelhardt contends that the failure of the Enlightenment was recapitulated by the secular proponents of bioethics starting in the 1960s as they attempted to provide "a rationally defensible ethics that can bind humans as such and justify in secular terms a content-rich account of human rights, duties, proper character, virtue,

[36] "The differences, however, have already become apparent, and it is no longer possible, if ever it was, to replace the soil and pretend they do not exist. They relate to the role of medicine and the doctor–patient relationship, to the proper methods of research and even the proper aims of research as well as to the familiar and more specific issues of abortion, euthanasia, and homosexuality. In the case of all of these, not far beneath the surface, will be found disagreements about the scope, character, and content of morality which in turn reflect more or less profound differences about the nature of human beings" (Mitchell, "The role of theology in bioethics," 65).

[37] H. Tristram Engelhardt, *The foundations of Christian bioethics* (Lisse: Swets & Zeitlinger, 2000), xii.

[38] Ibid., xi–3.

[39] Ibid., 24.

sentiments of care, etc."[40] But the pluralism that plagued Christianity after the Reformation similarly disrupts contemporary attempts to unify secular bioethics. According to Engelhardt, such attempts proceed as if a common moral background were available, discount the significance of moral disagreement or marginalize those who disagree with the reigning secular view, and generally refuse to allow space for disagreeing parties to pursue parallel moral visions.[41] Engelhardt believes that the denial of deep moral diversity is motivated by a desire to justify public policies that those in positions of power and influence wish to be dominant. A claim of a secular moral consensus is made to legitimize public policy, and in consequence a morally particular (not universal) bioethics becomes established despite persistent moral disagreements within society. Differences are denied so that the conclusions endorsed by official ethics commissions can be claimed to derive from a common morality believed to be recognized by all humans.[42] For Engelhardt, the outcome of the history of moral fracture is a deep pluralism in which individual persons, through the permission they grant to each other as morally autonomous selves, are the source of secular moral authority. "The question becomes which individuals have agreed to do what with whom."[43]

As a result of the deep pluralism that pervades society and bioethics, there is a socially pervasive focus on rights and due process, which in bioethics translates into the intense attention devoted to informed consent and the procedures by which decisions are reached rather than on the moral substance (goodness or badness) of choices made. This represents a shift to *proceduralism* in ethics, which Charles Taylor describes as manifesting itself in a preponderant concern with what is right to do rather than with what is good to be or to love.[44] The focus on procedure has left behind traditional understandings of the good life or the good as an object of our allegiance. Moral theory shaped by a proceduralist temperament emphasizes some criterion or other by which to derive obligatory actions. Kantians and utilitarians alike employ a proceduralist emphasis, either through universalization or maximizing calculation, respectively. In either case, substantive moral considerations are neglected in determining what constitutes pursuit of the good. Taylor believes the

40 Ibid., 25.
41 Ibid., 28.
42 Ibid., 29.
43 Ibid., 39.
44 Taylor, *Sources of the self*, 79.

stress on procedure is bound up with a modern allegiance to freedom,[45] and he notes that the principle of respect for persons has come to be expressed in terms of rights, thereby allowing the procedural to trump the substantive at the very center of moral concern.[46]

Taylor contends that the emphasis on procedure at the expense of substance has resulted in an ethics of inarticulacy regarding the deeper moral beliefs that support commitments to proceduralism. Despite their strong moral ideals – such as freedom and universalism – modern moral theorists "are constitutionally incapable of coming clean about the deeper sources of their own thinking."[47] They remain trapped by their insistence on the priority of the *right* over the *good*. They deprive themselves access to an articulation of the good that would provide meaning to the rules that define the right. Reference to the good has been suppressed, creating an inarticulacy about some of the most important concerns in ethics. "The strange cramped theories of modern moral philosophy . . . utterly mystify the priority of the moral by identifying it not with substance but with a form of reasoning, around which they draw a firm boundary."[48] Taylor considers this inarticulacy to be one of the roots of the "motivated suppression of moral ontology among our contemporaries," which he views as a reaction to having to grope for answers in the unanswered search for a basis for our moral intuitions.[49] The silence created by this suppression leaves perplexing gaps in contemporary ethical theory, caused by an inability to capture the background beliefs about the good that are fundamentally involved in our moral judgments.[50]

VI. MEDICAL PROFESSIONALS AND THE OBLIGATION TO PROVIDE CARE

The unique features of medical practice create special obligations for the physician, obligations that are of weighty importance when we consider

45 "To make practical reason substantive implies that practical wisdom is a matter of seeing an order which in some sense is in nature. This order determines what ought to be done. To reverse this and give primacy to the agent's own desires or his will, while still wanting to give value to practical reason, you have to redefine this in procedural terms. If the right thing to do still has to be understood as what is rationally justifiable, then the justification has to be procedural. It can't be defined by the particular outcome, but by the way in which the outcome is arrived at" (ibid., 85).

46 Ibid., 11.

47 Ibid., 88.

48 Ibid., 89.

49 Ibid., 10.

50 Ibid., 87.

the degree of freedom physicians should have to practice medicine according to their own understanding of what integrity entails. As citizens, physicians are like other individuals in society and deserve latitude to conduct their lives in keeping with their particular cultures, beliefs, and values in ways that are consistent with the requirements of a democratic society. But as professionals, physicians are more than citizens when it comes to questions of freedom and obligation in relation to patient care and public health. By entering the medical profession, they freely assume additional commitments, some of which are moral and some of which are defined by law. These additional commitments create obligations that determine professional responsibilities that may, to some extent, limit some of the freedoms they otherwise enjoy as citizens. It is important to consider the grounds that are usually considered to support the need to fulfill these obligations, for doing so can help us decide whether a physician's professional commitments should limit the expression of her individual beliefs and values (in word or deed), when doing so may conflict with social expectations. Three kinds of rationale are typically offered.

Respect for patient autonomy is perhaps the most common justification for claiming that physicians have an obligation to meet the needs and preferences of patients. This rationale may be voiced, for instance, by the claim that when a conscience-driven physician refuses to provide a treatment that is available and desired by a patient, that physician is imposing a constraint on her patient that is based on beliefs the patient does not share. The imposition of such a constraint, it is claimed, violates respect for the principle of autonomy "that holds that persons should be free to choose and act without controlling constraints imposed by others."[51] Though the principle of autonomy is only one of the guiding ethical principles in the practice of medicine, when it is invoked in debates about conscientious refusals by health professionals it is likely to be treated as having an importance that supersedes other ethical principles and values, whether beneficence (regarding the patient) or respect for conscience (regarding the professional). Closely related to claims focusing on patient autonomy are claims that the assessments of benefits and harms in a given scenario should not be controlled by professional judgment, but should ultimately depend on patients' perceptions of their own well-being.[52] It is also argued that special professional obligations derive from power differentials between physicians and patients, based on

[51] ACOG, "The limits of conscientious refusal in reproductive medicine."
[52] Ibid.

their respective differences in knowledge, skill, and health.[53] Attention to such differentials reflects a concern for the inherent inequalities between patients and physicians, as well as an awareness of the physician's professed obligation to restore the patient's humanity when it has been compromised by illness.[54]

A second rationale focuses on the voluntary nature of medical practice. Physicians enter their profession willingly and therefore should be, it is claimed, ready to assume all of the activities associated with their profession. Proponents of this view believe that because role-specific obligations are known and voluntarily accepted, it can be justifiable to limit physicians' claims of conscience, on the grounds that it is "unreasonable for an individual to enter a profession or specialty with primary activities that conflict with his or her central values."[55] Objections to such claims quickly arise regarding disagreements over which activities should be considered primary, and efforts to resolve such disputes inevitably bring one back to potentially contested questions about definitions of health and disease and the goals of medicine. Such fundamental questions underlie discussions of conscientious practice, and they ought to be engaged rather than sidestepped on the assumption that whatever practices are currently legal are morally required. Those who oppose conscientious refusals in some medical circumstances may attempt to draw a contrast between conscientious objection to military service and conscientious objection within the health professions, based on the involuntary nature of military conscription and the voluntary nature of professional practice.[56] But such a comparison presumes that the military and the medical profession are similar regarding the degree to which their required activities are coherent with their stated goals. The conscientious objector to military service typically objects to the military's primary commitment to use lethal force as a means to defend national interests. By contrast, the conscientious objector to certain practices within the health professions does not object to the professions' primary commitment to use scientific knowledge and

53 AAP, "Policy statement."

54 Edmund D. Pellegrino, *Humanism and the physician* (Knoxville: University of Tennessee Press, 1979), 123.

55 AAP, "Policy statement."

56 "Conscientious objection makes sense with conscription, but it is worrisome when professionals who freely choose their field parse care and withhold information that patients need. As the gatekeepers to medicine, physicians and other health care providers have an obligation to choose specialties that are not moral minefields for them." Cantor, "Conscientious objection gone awry," 1485.

clinical skills as means to promote health and healing. Rather, the question for the conscientious health care professional is whether a given practice promotes health and healing, not whether scientific knowledge and clinical skills should generally be used as means to health and healing.

A third type of justification that may be claimed for limiting conscientious objection by physicians is based on social expectations. This rationale is consistent with the belief that medicine should be understood as a socially constructed practice, and it holds that society is entitled to expect physicians to practice according to accepted roles and standards of care, which are shaped by a wide range of professional, institutional, legal, and market influences. Some who support this rationale believe that constraints on conscience are justifiable because a physician has a duty to fulfill an exclusive social role that is protected by the monopolizing privileges of professional licensure.[57] Others see this rationale as part of medical professionalism, on the belief that "professionalism entails actions that are required of physicians to meet the expectations of patients and the public,"[58] that "civic professionalism" must sustain the relationship between medicine and society in order to promote the common good,[59] and that physicians serve as "guardians of social values" and are expected to respond to society's needs.[60] This professional responsibility to satisfy social expectations may at times be framed in terms of what is legally permissible, on the assumption that physicians have a moral responsibility to provide, or support the provision of, any service that is legal.[61]

VII. OBLIGATION AND INDEPENDENCE IN THE "SOCIAL CONTRACT" BETWEEN MEDICINE AND SOCIETY

The social expectations just described can be seen as part of a "social contract" between society and the medical profession, a contract that is

57 AAP, "Policy statement."

58 Jordan J. Cohen, "Linking professionalism to humanism: what it means, why it matters," *Academic Medicine* 82 (2007): 1029–32.

59 W. M. Sullivan, "Medicine under threat: professionalism and professional identity," *Canadian Medical Association Journal* 162 (2000): 673–75.

60 Herbert M. Swick, "Toward a normative definition of medical professionalism," *Academic Medicine* 75 (2000): 612–16.

61 "Physicians should support an ethic that allows for all legal options, even those they would not choose. Federal laws may make room for the rights of conscience, but health care providers – and all those whose jobs affect patient care – should cast off the cloak of conscience when patients' needs demand it." Cantor, "Conscientious objection gone awry," 1485.

mutually demanding and beneficial. On the one hand, society grants the medical profession a substantial degree of autonomy, self-regulation, and monopolistic control, as well as high levels of compensation and esteem. On the other hand, society expects physicians to be altruistic, competent, ethical, and committed to advancing the public good by meeting the medical needs of society.[62] The contract is composed of a wide range of reciprocal expectations and obligations, many of which are formalized or mandated through laws, regulation, licensing, and professional certification. At its core is the expectation that a physician will fulfill his healing role through altruistic service, respect for patient autonomy, promotion of the public good, and a commitment to ethical values and integrity – and the primary place where this fiduciary role is fulfilled is in the care of individual patients.[63] The professional obligation represented by the social contract is sufficiently weighty that some claim the medical profession has a responsibility to provide "all legal and beneficial medical interventions sought by patients" because "a profession's responsibilities are to the society it serves and by which it is licensed and regulated, and the determination of those responsibilities is not within the sole authority of the profession."[64] Some go so far as to suggest that by granting the medical profession a monopoly on medical services, society turns medicine "into a kind of public utility, obligated to provide service to all who seek it."[65]

As established and extensive as the social contract is, we should not view it as proof that the essence of medicine is determined by social expectations. As discussed in Chapter 1, there are contrasting ways to identify the sources of value that ought to determine how medicine should be practiced, one of which is the social constructivist position. On this view, medicine's goals will vary across times and cultures, depending on the values and priorities of a given society. But social expectations are not the only sources of value at play. Medicine is also influenced by concepts of health and disease, professional judgments about the values most appropriate to promote health and healing, and the internal goods of medical practice that dictate goals that are independent of a society's externally

[62] Richard L. Cruess and Sylvia R. Cruess, "Expectations and obligations: professionalism and medicine's social contract with society," *Perspectives in Biology and Medicine* 51, no. 4 (2008): 579–98.

[63] Ibid.

[64] Brock, "Conscientious refusal by physicians and pharmacists."

[65] Charo, "The celestial fire of conscience."

imposed purposes and reflect enduring and universal responses to the human experience of illness.[66]

The disagreement between a socially constructed view and an internally or professionally guided view is reflected in a parallel disagreement about how the social contract should be interpreted. An interpretation that favors greater degrees of control on physicians would see physicians as civil servants bound to provide all legally available services to patients who request them. By contrast, an interpretation that favors greater degrees of physician autonomy would see physicians as recognizing certain social obligations while also maintaining that socially determined obligations are not independent of, or superior to, the goals that physicians take to be intrinsic to the practice of medicine. Those who hold to a more autonomy-respecting interpretation would see physicians as moral agents whose convictions – derived from professional and individual beliefs – serve as an interpretive framework by which medicine's intrinsic and social purposes are understood and by which its obligations to society are decided. Evidence suggests that many physicians in the United States may have views that resonate with both kinds of interpretations, given that 77 percent believe they have the right to refuse to provide legal medical procedures if they believe those procedures are morally wrong and 82 percent believe that when they do refuse to provide a legally available service they must refer patients to another physician who will provide the service.[67]

The tension between society's prerogative to impose its will on medicine and the medical professional's prerogative to exercise independent judgment invites us to look for perspectives on the patient–physician relationship that acknowledge the existence of controversial areas of practice and provide space for conscientious practice within those areas. Mark Siegler has articulated a vision of the patient–physician relationship that provides this kind of space through what he calls the doctor–patient accommodation, based on his belief that the patient–physician encounter requires a negotiated accommodation between two individuals in order to achieve mutually satisfactory goals.[68] This accommodation depends on the particularities of both the patient and the physician (regarding personality, character, attitude, values, and, for the physician, technical

[66] Hanson and Callahan, *The goals of medicine*, 15–16.

[67] Ryan E. Lawrence and Farr A. Curlin, "Physicians' beliefs about conscience in medicine: a national survey," *Academic Medicine* 84 (2009): 1276–82.

[68] Siegler, "The doctor–patient encounter and its relationship to theories of health and disease."

skills), on trust and mutual consent, and on a balance between the needs of the patient and the standards of the medical profession as understood by the physician. The values that guide the physician are derived both from professional training and from moral commitments that precede it. For Siegler, the physician's beliefs and values are important enough to warrant the protection of conscientious behavior within the doctor–patient accommodation, with the result that the physician is not obligated to participate in practices she believes to be illegal, immoral, or outside the bounds of medical care.

Siegler's approach emphasizes the value of mutuality in the patient–physician relationship. When framed in terms of mutual respect, this relationship can be seen as requiring bilateral respect for moral agency.[69] On such an account, one of the things patients expect when seeking care from physicians is respect for their personal autonomy, including the freedom to refuse treatment. And one of the things physicians expect is respect for their integrity, including the freedom to refuse to participate in a service when there are serious grounds for moral objection. This bilateral respect for moral agency may also be characterized in terms of rights, which can serve as a reminder that a medical professional should never be viewed merely as a function of her socially mandated role, but always also as a person in herself who maintains certain basic freedoms.

VIII. SUMMARY

Among some observers of bioethics, there is concern that references to religious beliefs are discouraged and that beliefs and values articulated in nonreligious terms are privileged. Assuming such concerns have at least some validity, resistance to religious references in medical and bioethical contexts can be seen as part of a wider opposition to the articulation of religious beliefs in political dialogues in liberal democracies. Such opposition claims that religious beliefs, when offered as reasons for laws or policies, do not satisfy the requirement of being accessible to "public reason." The motivation behind this concern for accessibility arises from the conviction that because political power is coercive, it is acceptable only when justified in terms accessible to the persons who are coerced. On such a view, the criterion of accessibility provides a basis for distinguishing

69 Robin Fretwell Wilson, "The limits of conscience: moral clashes over deeply divisive healthcare procedures," *American Journal of Law & Medicine* 34, (2008): 41–63.

between public moral reasons that are politically relevant and private religious reasons that are not.

For Rawls, modern democratic society is characterized by a pluralism of incompatible yet reasonable comprehensive doctrines, which may be religious, political, or moral. These doctrines somehow need to coexist and support the political conception of a constitutional democracy. He proposed a conception of political justice that a plurality of reasonable doctrines might endorse, defined by an overlapping consensus that is independent of all comprehensive doctrines but still sustained by the capacity of those doctrines for deeper and fuller moral justification. He believed this overlapping consensus could be acknowledged by all citizens on the basis of public reason, which is constituted by presently accepted general beliefs, commonsense reasoning, and scientific reasoning. For Rawls, public reason was the necessary common denominator for legitimate political dialogue. Religious or other comprehensive beliefs could be introduced into political discourse, but only if public reasons for principles and policies were also provided.

Habermas believes the Rawlsian separation of religious and secular language imposes an asymmetrical burden on people of religious faith, causing cognitive dissonance when they are compelled to act publicly as if religious beliefs could be set aside in the public sphere. Habermas holds that such persons should not be expected to divide their identity into public and private components and that political dialogue entails a shared responsibility for the translation of ideas between secular and religious persons. Like Rawls, Habermas would prohibit religious expression and justification among lawmakers and policy makers in the absence of a parallel justification expressed in secular terms; but unlike Rawls, he supports religious expression in the public square by ordinary citizens.

By contrast, Wolterstorff objects to the epistemic basis of the Rawlsian position, arguing that its restraints on religious beliefs in public arguments are mistakenly premised on the assumption that religious beliefs, to be valid, must be of a certain sort and compatible with presumptions about common rationality. Contrary to Rawls, Wolterstorff maintains that we are endowed with belief dispositions that give rise to *immediate* beliefs that make rationality *situated*, such that our beliefs are rational unless we have reasons for refraining from believing them. This implies that religious convictions need not be reinforced by supposedly more fundamental beliefs to be valid in public. Wolterstorff believes that Rawls's idea of public reason fails to respect people's need to think and live in ways that express the religious or other comprehensive beliefs that define their lives and require integration with their choices and actions. To Wolterstorff, Rawls's entire project suffers from a misplaced attempt to discover a shared political basis for a communitarian politics and an unwillingness to accept the need to live within a politics defined by multiple moral-religious communities. If Wolterstorff's assessment is accurate, the notion of public reason is overstated, since all rationality is situated. As a result, reasoning that refers to comprehensive beliefs should not automatically be dismissed from the public square. Instead of postulating the existence of public reason, we should see the need to live in a world of diverse reasons, contested policies, and deliberated compromises that form the conditions of a morally pluralistic and stable democracy.

Another reason to allow space for the expression of religious belief in professional and public discourse is based on the fundamentally dialogical character of moral life. As Taylor describes, we understand ourselves morally through our dialogues with other persons, not in individualistic isolation. Our moral identities are cultivated through communication with others, and the act of articulating our moral beliefs and reasons empowers us to pursue what we believe is good. As individuals articulate their reasons for living an integrated life, their listeners are informed, their own reasons are opened to critical reflection, and their moral identities are strengthened.

While the debate about the place of religious beliefs in the public square tends to be engaged in reference to citizens and/or public officials, we should ask whether medical professionals should be viewed more as ordinary citizens (and given more latitude) or as public officials (and given less latitude) in the course of their professional activities. The answer to this question depends on one's assessment of the obligations of a medical professional. By entering the medical profession, physicians assume specific commitments that create special professional responsibilities that may impose restrictions on individual freedom. But the justifications for such restrictions remain open to debate because of uncertainties surrounding important questions, such as the relative importance of patient autonomy and professional autonomy, controversies over what should be considered a medical service, and the extent to which freedom of conscience should be honored.

The obligations of medical professionals are often examined in terms of a "social contract" between society and the medical profession, in which society grants the profession special privileges and in return expects certain benefits. Some favor an interpretation of the contract that exerts greater degrees of control on physicians, adopting a social constructivist view of the medical profession that claims physicians are properly viewed as civil servants and obligated to provide all legally available medical services. But others favor an interpretation that provides a greater degree of physician autonomy, viewing professionals as guardians of a practice who are entitled to establish boundaries of professional obligation based on professional and individual beliefs – beliefs that serve as a framework for interpreting medicine's intrinsic and social purposes, especially when debatable concepts of health and disease pertain to controversial medical services. The tension between society's prerogative to impose its will on medicine and the medical professional's prerogative to exercise independent judgment invites us to look for more nuanced visions of the relationship between patients and medical professionals. Such visions ought to acknowledge the pervasiveness of moral pluralism, reflect the existence of controversial areas of practice, and provide space for conscientious practice – especially at the level of the patient–physician relationship, where the bilateral moral agency of patients and physicians should be honored through mutual respect and freedom.

9

Conscientious Objection and Conscientious Practice

In recent years a considerable amount of attention has been focused on the tensions that arise when physicians and other health care professionals refuse to provide certain legally available services because of objections based on professional, moral, or religious beliefs and values. These conscientious objections are often interpreted as representing a conflict between the personal beliefs of a health professional and the medical needs of a patient. On such views, conscientious objections represent a conflict with society's expectation that medical services ought to be provided whenever they are legal, available, and requested. The extent of the challenge posed by conscientious objections can be seen in the results of two surveys of U.S. physicians regarding controversial medical practices. One of these documented that (only) 71 percent of physicians believe they are obligated to refer patients to another clinician who does not object to a controversial procedure that has been requested, and (only) 86 percent believe they are obligated to present all treatment options to patients when controversial clinical practices are at issue.[1] Another study found that (only) 57 percent of physicians agreed that doctors must refer patients to other clinicians for all legally available medical services regardless of whether the referring physician believes the referral itself is immoral.[2]

Those who question the legitimacy of conscientious objections usually believe physicians have an obligation to provide or facilitate access to services that are considered medical. They may also interpret the

[1] Farr A. Curlin et al., "Religion, conscience, and controversial clinical practices," *New England Journal of Medicine* 356 (2007): 593–600.

[2] Michael P. Combs et al., "Conscientious refusals to refer: findings from a national physician survey," *Journal of Medical Ethics* 37 (2011): 397–401.

unwillingness to fulfill this obligation as an imposition of the physician's beliefs on the patient – thereby violating patient autonomy. One of the central concerns of this chapter is to question whether the unwillingness to provide or facilitate access to services deemed objectionable should be viewed in this way. In addressing this concern, I assume that an assessment of this issue should take into consideration the potentially competing claims of three parties – patients, physicians, and society – so that the relative merits of their claims can be weighed. Along with a consideration of these claims, there is a need to consider two other issues. First, attention should be given to the basis upon which a service is defined as "medical," since a medical designation itself can suggest a presumptive obligation for physicians, which may or may not be justified. Second, it is important to appreciate the moral difference between nonparticipation (e.g., when a physician refuses to cooperate with a patient's intentions) and interference (e.g., when a physician endeavors to thwart a patient's intentions).

Various individuals and organizations have made recommendations or offered guidelines for managing conscientious refusals in a way that balances the interests of patients, physicians, and society. These recommendations are directed primarily toward physicians and other health care professionals but may also be directed toward the institutions that employ them. The content of the recommendations typically involves one or more duties: to disclose information (by giving prior notice, describing alternatives, and explaining the reasons for refusal), to facilitate treatment (by referring or transferring care to another health care professional), to provide treatment (in cases of emergency or when other means of treatment are unavailable), or to avoid undertaking professional work that includes activities to which one objects (by avoiding specialty areas of medicine that are perceived as problematic, by eschewing the medical profession entirely if its problematic areas are too widespread, or by quitting the profession if its service demands are realized only after one has entered the profession). This chapter begins with a description of these proposed duties, along with examples from organizations or individuals who support them.

I. PROFESSIONAL DUTIES THAT MIGHT BE SAID TO PLACE LIMITS ON CONSCIENTIOUS OBJECTION IN MEDICINE

A. Duty to Give Prior Notice

The duty to inform patients in advance about potential restrictions of health care services is widely supported. For example, the American

Academy of Pediatrics (AAP) holds that physicians have "a duty to prospective patients to disclose standard treatments and procedures that they refuse to provide but are normally provided by other health care professionals."[3] The American Congress of Obstetrics and Gynecology (ACOG) likewise holds that when "conscience implores physicians to deviate from standard practices, including abortion, sterilization, and provision of contraceptives, they must provide potential patients with accurate and prior notice of their personal moral commitments."[4] Some writers believe that giving prior notice to prospective patients and prospective employers should be a minimum expectation for physicians with conscientious objections to certain services[5] and that physicians and institutions would be well advised to make such policies known to patients.[6] Others stress the need to disclose such information to persons after they have been accepted as patients[7] but in advance of crisis situations.[8] Concerns about the duty to give prior notice have led to laws that require managed care and insurance plans to inform potential enrollees of services that are not covered because of the religious beliefs of practitioners.[9]

B. Duty to Inform about Alternatives

It is also widely held that physicians who are unwilling to provide a medical service within their specialty's scope of practice have a duty to inform patients of alternative means of securing that service. The AAP believes that this duty is part of the informed consent process,[10] the ACOG refers to it as a duty of disclosing information necessary for patients to make informed decisions,[11] and the American College of Physicians (ACP) holds that an objecting physician "has a duty to inform the patient about care options and alternatives, or refer the patient for such information, so that

[3] AAP, "Policy statement."

[4] ACOG, "The limits of conscientious refusal in reproductive medicine."

[5] Beauchamp and Childress, *Principles of biomedical ethics*, 45.

[6] J. David Bleich, "The physician as a conscientious objector," *Fordham Urban Law Journal* 30 (2002): 245–65.

[7] B. M. Dickens and R. J. Cook, "The scope and limits of conscientious objection," *International Journal of Gynecology & Obstetrics* 71 (2000): 71–77.

[8] Pellegrino, "The physician's conscience, conscience clauses, and religious belief."

[9] Katherine A. White, "Crisis of conscience: reconciling religious health care providers' beliefs and patients' rights," *Stanford Law Review* 51 (1999): 1703–49.

[10] AAP, "Policy statement."

[11] ACOG, "The limits of conscientious refusal in reproductive medicine."

the patient's rights are not constrained."[12] Various authors echo these statements when writing that physicians "always have an ethical duty to disclose options for obtaining legal, albeit morally controversial, services,"[13] that informing patients about services relevant to their condition is part of the "conventional compromise" that accommodates conscientious objection,[14] that patients need all legal alternatives explained,[15] and that a system of counseling should be accessible so that all patients have the information needed to make their own decisions.[16] Such commentators view information about treatment alternatives as a minimum level of duty.

C. Duty to Inform about Reasons for Refusal

Another area of information that some believe is important for disclosure is the rationale behind a physician's objection to a medical service. Such writers argue that professionals motivated by religious objections should reveal their motivations to avoid misleading patients about the reasons for not pursuing a possible course of treatment.[17] Otherwise, patients may be under the false impression that medical – rather than moral – reasons are guiding a recommendation and potentially limiting knowledge of treatment options.[18]

D. Duty to Refer to Another Practitioner or Facility

There is also a frequently expressed belief that objecting physicians have a duty to refer patients to another professional who is presumed to be willing to provide the service at issue. The AAP and the ACOG believe that physicians have a duty to refer patients "in a timely manner,"[19] and the ACP likewise affirms the need for referral to ensure that relevant information about treatment options is disclosed.[20] The American Medical Association (AMA) provides a similar recommendation, albeit one that

[12] ACP, *American College of Physicians ethics manual*, 6th ed. (Philadelphia, 2012).

[13] Beauchamp and Childress, *Principles of biomedical ethics*, 45.

[14] Brock, "Conscientious refusal by physicians and pharmacists."

[15] Cantor, "Conscientious objection gone awry."

[16] Charo, "The celestial fire of conscience."

[17] Minow, "On being a religious professional."

[18] John K. Davis, "Conscientious refusal and a doctor's right to quit," *Journal of Medicine and Philosophy* 29 (2004): 75–91.

[19] AAP, "Policy statement"; ACOG, "The limits of conscientious refusal in reproductive medicine."

[20] ACP, *American College of Physicians ethics manual*.

allows for exceptions: "a conscientious objection should, under most circumstances, be accompanied by a referral to another physician or health care facility."[21] A similarly qualified stance on the need for referrals is communicated by those who believe that referral is necessary "in many cases,"[22] or that the need for referral depends on "the presence or lack of ethical consensus within the profession,"[23] or that referral is needed so long as the requested procedure "is not sufficiently immoral to justify interference" with a patient's choice.[24] However, there are also those who believe that a referral may not be a legitimate alternative to the provision of care if a referral imposes "an unreasonable burden on the patient."[25] Other assessments take a collective view of professionals, claiming that a health profession should create mechanisms that allow patients to work around the objections of an individual clinician by means of institutional policies and procedures,[26] professional referral systems,[27] or open and direct access to desired services under insurance plans[28] – thereby placing the responsibility for providing access to care on an entire profession rather than on any one of its members.

E. Duty to Transfer Care

Closely related to referrals are claims regarding the duty to transfer care; sometimes these two concerns are taken together or are treated as interchangeable.[29] However, whereas a referral may only require providing information about alternative means of care in a given case, a transfer of care is a formal action that is not only permitted by a patient but also authorized by two professionals, one of whom "sends" and one of whom "receives" the patient. Nuance in discussions of transfers is evidenced by the way some authors speak of a physician's duty to "undertake the transfer" of patients she is unwilling to treat,[30] while others describe the patient's "right

[21] AMA, Council on Judicial Affairs, "Physician objection to treatment and individual patient discrimination" (CEJA report no. 6-A-07) (American Medical Association, 2007).
[22] Beauchamp and Childress, *Principles of biomedical ethics*, 45.
[23] Blustein, "Doing what the patient orders."
[24] Davis, "Conscientious refusal and a doctor's right to quit."
[25] Brock, "Conscientious refusal by physicians and pharmacists."
[26] Combs et al., "Conscientious refusals to refer"; Wilson, "The limits of conscience."
[27] Charo, "The celestial fire of conscience."
[28] White, "Crisis of conscience."
[29] ACP, *American College of Physicians ethics manual*; Combs et al., "Conscientious refusals to refer."
[30] Dickens and Cook, "The scope and limits of conscientious objection."

to seek transfer" to another health care facility.[31] This indicates how a transfer of care can be seen as either a physician's obligation or a patient's prerogative. In any case, a transfer of care requires the active cooperation of the objecting physician.

F. Duty to Treat

It may also be claimed that objecting physicians have a duty to provide controversial treatments in cases of emergency or when an alternative means of treatment is unavailable or inaccessible. The AAP, for example, believes that physicians have a moral obligation to provide treatment "when referral would significantly increase the probability of mortality or serious morbidity" and that the duty to treat "increases as the availability of alternative providers decreases and the risk to the patient increases."[32] Likewise, the ACOG believes that in emergent situations involving a patient's physical or mental health, "providers have an obligation to provide medically indicated and requested care regardless of the provider's personal moral objections" and, more generally, that physicians are obligated to treat patients when there are no other "resources in place to allow the patient to gain access to care."[33]

G. Duty to Avoid Activities to Which One Objects

Some commentators believe that individuals should not enter the medical profession, or a specialty area within it, if doing so would most likely pose conflicts of conscience related to some of the services that are part of the profession or one of its specialties. Some would add that persons who come to realize that such a conflict exists after entry into the medical profession should see the option of quitting the profession as a potentially necessary concession. Such views trade on beliefs about voluntariness that emphasize the freedom with which physicians enter their profession and accept a duty to provide care. Writers of this persuasion hold that physicians who are unwilling to provide legally available and specialty-appropriate care or who insist on referring patients elsewhere for it should

[31] Bleich, "The physician as a conscientious objector."
[32] AAP, "Policy statement."
[33] ACOG, "The limits of conscientious refusal in reproductive medicine."

find alternative work within their profession that poses no conflicts or, if that is not possible, leave the profession entirely.[34]

II. TWO POSSIBLE STANDARDS FOR CALIBRATING THE ACCEPTABLE RANGE OF CONSCIENTIOUS OBJECTION

The recommendations offered by various organizations and individuals regarding the extent to which conscientious objections should be tolerated among physicians can be considered according to the way different values are prioritized. On the one hand, there are those who apply what I would call a *physician-regulating standard,* which places first priority on a patient's right to request and receive medical services that are legal and available, such that the value of a physician's conscience may need to be subordinated to this patient right. On the other hand, there are those who apply what I would call a *physician-respecting standard,* which acknowledges the physician's prima facie obligation to respect and promote patients' treatment preferences, while also recognizing that a professional's conscience merits an essential measure of respect and protection. (The difference between these standards parallels the contrasting interpretations of the social contract discussed in Chapter 8.) Both standards are socially determined, that is, based on existing laws and professional standards of care, and both standards are patient-oriented, that is, based on the need to respect a patient's freedom to make his own decisions. But the difference between them comes into play when questions of professional conscience arise. A physician-regulating standard presumes that society has the prerogative to determine what services physicians must – for moral reasons – provide or facilitate. A physician-respecting standard presumes that physicians have the prerogative to determine what services they are unable – for moral reasons – to provide or facilitate. A physician-regulating standard tilts the ethical priority toward socially approved patient preferences, whereas the physician-respecting standard tilts the ethical priority toward professional integrity. A physician-regulating standard would support laws and policies that increase the uniformity of medical practice by reserving *less* space for conscientious objection. A physician-respecting standard would support laws and policies that protect *more* space for conscientious objection and thereby increase opportunities for physicians to express their moral integrity in medical practice.

[34] Brock, "Conscientious refusal by physicians and pharmacists"; Minow, "On being a religious professional"; Savulescu, "Conscientious objection in medicine."

A. Examples of a Physician-Regulating Standard

Positions representing a physician-regulating standard can be found in the statements of major medical organizations and among individual commentators. The ACOG, for instance, concludes that "ethical care requires either that the physician provide care despite reservations or that there be resources in place to allow the patient to gain access to care in the presence of conscientious refusal."[35] This position is based on the belief that a patient's health-related interests supersede what are viewed as a physician's personal interests pertaining to conscience. Respect for conscience, according to the ACOG, "is only a prima facie value, which means it can and should be overridden in the interest of other moral obligations that outweigh it in a given circumstance." The ACOG portrays conscience as a "personal interest" that must yield to patient autonomy by force of the duties physicians accept upon entering the medical profession. Similarly, the ACP believes that a physician, though not obligated to recommend, perform, or prescribe services he finds objectionable, nevertheless "has a duty to inform the patient about care options and alternatives, or refer the patient for such information," and if he is unable to provide such information should transfer a patient's care.[36] The ACP bases this position on the belief that a physician has an ethical duty to disclose relevant information about medical services and that a physician's individual moral standards should not be allowed to constrain the rights of a patient to receive information about, and access to, treatment.

Some organizations and individual writers who adopt a physician-regulating standard also mark the need for institutional mechanisms to accommodate physicians who refuse to provide certain services because of their conscientious objections. The AAP, for instance, recommends that employers provide reasonable accommodations for objecting physicians, even as they join the ACOG and the ACP in holding that physicians have obligations to inform, refer, and provide emergency treatment. The AAP views reasonable accommodation as a way to promote the protection of physician conscience while ensuring the provision of legal services.[37] Beauchamp and Childress also support physician accommodations, so long as patients' rights and interests are not compromised.[38] Others

[35] ACOG, "The limits of conscientious refusal in reproductive medicine."

[36] ACP, *American College of Physicians ethics manual.*

[37] AAP, "Policy statement."

[38] Beauchamp and Childress, *Principles of biomedical ethics*, 44–45.

concur, recognizing that antidiscrimination law obligates employers to provide reasonable accommodations for conscientious refusals by physicians, so long as patients' interests are protected.[39]

Another example of the physician-regulating standard can be found in the work of Mark Wicclair. He acknowledges the need to promote moral integrity among physicians and accommodate their appeals to conscience whenever possible, so long as this does not compromise patients' rights and interests.[40] His argument for accommodation is particularly sensitive to the need to protect conscience when objections are based on a physician's self-conception as an ethical professional. However, the need for accommodation is less warranted if claims of conscience arise from other identities a physician may have, based on religious, ethnic, or cultural affiliations. With this distinction, he suggests a separation of a physician's "professional" and "personal" identities, thereby questioning a notion of moral integrity in which the "professional" and "personal" would be seen as genuinely integrated. Wicclair's willingness to subordinate the conscientious objections of physicians to the rights of patients can also be seen in the way he prioritizes three core professional obligations: to respect patient dignity and refrain from discrimination, promote patient health and well-being, and respect patient autonomy.[41] He believes that these obligations justify the placement of limits on the exercise of a physician's conscience in relation to five areas (the last three of which depend on the circumstances at hand): discrimination; patient harms and burdens; disclosing options; referral and/or facilitating a transfer; and advance notification.[42]

Another possible manifestation of a physician-regulating standard is evidenced by writers who believe that physicians have an obligation to abandon professional roles that carry expectations for socially approved and professionally accepted medical services to which they object. Brock, for instance, maintains that physicians should be willing to balance their professional obligations with their individual moral integrity by informing and referring patients, and if they are unwilling to do so, they should remove themselves from practice settings that occasion conscientious refusals.[43] Likewise, Minow believes that if conflicts between professionals

39 Dickens and Cook, "The scope and limits of conscientious objection."

40 Wicclair, "Conscientious objection in medicine."

41 Mark R. Wicclair, *Conscientious objection in health care: an ethical analysis* (Cambridge: Cambridge University Press, 2011), 88.

42 Ibid., 92.

43 Brock, "Conscientious refusal by physicians and pharmacists."

and patients due to deeply held beliefs cannot be managed by referrals or other means to meet the needs of patients, clinicians should move away from controversial practice environments or abandon their professional roles entirely.[44]

Finally, some of those who promote a physician-regulating standard assume that the extent of a physician's professional obligation can be determined by the domain of legally available services. Savulescu adopts this view, suggesting that professional conscience "has little place in the delivery of modern medical care" because what patients should receive from physicians is defined by law, standards of just distribution of health care resources, and "a reasonable conception of the patient's good and the patient's informed desires." He claims that persons unwilling to offer legally permitted services should not be physicians, and physicians "who compromise the delivery of medical services to patients on conscience grounds must be punished through removal of license to practice and other legal mechanisms."[45]

B. Examples of a Physician-Respecting Standard

Positions reflecting a physician-respecting standard do not appear to be common among major medical organizations, but they can be found among individual commentators on conscientious objection or related considerations. These commentators place a high premium on protecting a professional's conscience while also promoting patient autonomy. They do so in ways that reflect the assumptions Childress makes when he writes, in reference to appeals to conscience generally speaking, that it "is prima facie a moral evil to force a person to act against his conscience," that "we should start with the presumptive liberty of conscience," and that the state should "bear the burden of proof to show that its interests are compelling and can be realized through no other means than a denial of the exemption [to conscientious objectors]."[46]

By recognizing that a professional's conscience merits an essential measure of respect and protection, versions of a physician-respecting standard favor a broader professional space in which physicians can practice medicine according to their conscience-based convictions. This broader professional space receives support from a range of arguments

44 Minow, "On being a religious professional," 685.
45 Savulescu, "Conscientious objection in medicine."
46 Childress, "Appeals to conscience."

pertaining to the nature of the patient–physician relationship and the freedoms and rights that pertain to patients and physicians. Thomas May offers two arguments in favor of such broader professional space.[47] The first distinguishes between objections to the *type* of treatment in question versus objections to a patient's evaluation of the *benefits and burdens* of that treatment: May maintains that although patients should have the right to assess the benefits and burdens of potential treatments for themselves, they should not have the right to demand any treatment they want. The second argument distinguishes between a *refusal* of treatment and a *request* for treatment: May maintains that although patients have the negative right to refuse treatment (i.e., the right to be left alone), they do not have a positive right to receive everything they may request. Daniel Sulmasy offers a different kind of rationale for a broader professional space for conscience, based on the relationship between conscience and tolerance. He views conscience as the fundamental commitment to be moral, a commitment that includes a respect for others that entails tolerating their exercise of conscience. In short, he suggests that tolerance is the mutual respect for conscience.[48]

The physician-respecting standard for conscience is also supported by conceptions of the patient–physician relationship that recognize a professional's freedom to determine the appropriate purposes of the relationship and to decide when to enter into it with a specific patient. Mark Siegler highlights the importance of this professional freedom in his discussion of the mutual accommodation that should occur in the patient–physician relationship. This accommodation includes the physician's determination of which goals and services are appropriate, based on the physician's "concept of professional standards and norms of behavior for physicians."[49] Siegler also believes a physician should not be required to abandon his own "standards of conscientious behavior to engage in illegal or immoral practices, to act in ways contrary to his own perception of what it is to be a good physician, or to participate in practices he believes to be outside of the legitimate medical sphere." Moreover, the values upon which a physician's perceptions are based should be expected to be a mixture of those adopted in medical training and those that existed prior to that training and still endure. Siegler's view

47 Thomas May, "Rights of conscience in health care," *Social Theory and Practice* 27 (2001): 111–28.

48 Sulmasy, "What is conscience and why is respect for it so important?"

49 Siegler, "The doctor–patient encounter and its relationship to theories of health and disease."

resonates with one of the core themes of this book – that all physicians have foundational beliefs that guide their thinking about medicine and ethics, beliefs that represent an integration of the values they bring to medicine and the values they learn through medical training and practice.

The professional freedom to guide the purposes of the physician–patient relationship is an established position of the AMA, according to which physicians should have the prerogative to decide whether to enter into a professional relationship with a given patient – except in situations constituting a medical emergency, involving discrimination, or falling under a contractual arrangement. According to the AMA's view of professional freedom, it may be "ethically permissible" for a physician to decline a potential patient when a desired treatment "is incompatible with the physician's personal, religious, or moral beliefs."[50] The AMA *Code of Medical Ethics* does not directly address how a physician should handle situations of such incompatibility after a relationship with a patient already exists. However, in a report by the AMA's Council on Ethical and Judicial Affairs (CEJA) in 2007, it was noted that the Code "makes clear that physicians may choose whom to serve," that "except in emergencies, they may refuse to provide a treatment to which they object on the basis of religious or moral beliefs," and that "other Principles balance this prerogative with obligations to respect patients and their ability to access available medical care," such that "a conscientious objection should, under most circumstances, be accompanied by a referral to another physician or health care facility."[51] The *Code of Medical Ethics* and this CEJA report taken together suggest that the AMA supports a physician-respecting standard for conscience, even as it also signals appreciation for a physician-regulating standard by recommending referrals in most circumstances.

By taking integrity seriously, the physician-respecting standard can be interpreted as reflecting the conviction that we should respect the autonomy of patients and physicians alike. This conviction is articulated by Pellegrino, when he maintains that neither the patient nor the physician is entitled to override the conscience of the other.[52] Framed in terms of negative rights, this conviction represents a certain symmetry, or equality, in which neither the patient nor the physician should be forced by the other to participate in decisions or actions that either considers morally

[50] AMA, Code of Medical Ethics, "Opinion 10.05: potential patients" (2008); www.ama-assn.org/ama/pub/physician-resources/medical-ethics/code-medical-ethics/opinion1005.page.

[51] AMA, "Physician objection to treatment and individual patient discrimination."

[52] Pellegrino, "The physician's conscience, conscience clauses, and religious belief."

objectionable. On such a view, a patient has a right not to be treated that is paralleled by a physician's right not to participate in treatment. Some may object that a patient and a physician cannot be viewed as equals in a relationship defined by asymmetries in health, knowledge, and power. This is a valid concern. One response to this concern is to acknowledge the need for prior disclosure, so that patients know in advance of a crisis whether certain treatments or services are unacceptable to certain physicians. But granting the existence of asymmetry in the patient–physician relationship does not settle the question of how freedom of conscience (i.e., mutual respect for moral autonomy) should be handled between patients and physicians. Although the asymmetry between patients and physicians justifies placing special moral and legal obligations on physicians, these obligations may find their proper limits at the point where a professional's conscience is violated. Taking integrity seriously provides a basis for such limits. And it is such a basis that underlies the conscience clauses in law that protect professionals who refuse, on grounds of conscience, to participate in services that are legally permitted but morally objectionable.

III. CONSCIENCE CLAUSES IN LAW TO PROTECT CONSCIENTIOUS OBJECTION

In the United States, conscience clauses arose initially in response to the legalization of abortion, and they currently exist in federal and most state laws.[53] The purpose of a conscience clause is to offer "explicit protection for the rights of health care providers to decline to provide or participate in providing health services that violate their religious or moral beliefs."[54] These protections stipulate the conditions under which individuals or organizations are legally entitled to space for conscientious objection to activities in which they would otherwise be obligated to participate. Though these protections have been contested, their need arises from a broadly shared belief that conscience represents a uniquely important feature of human existence that deserves to be protected by government guarantees.[55] Furthermore, they reflect our recognition that some public

[53] Wilson, "The limits of conscience."

[54] Lynn D. Wardle, "Protecting the rights of conscience of health care providers," *Journal of Legal Medicine* 14 (1993): 177–230.

[55] Nussbaum, *Liberty of conscience*, 19–20.

policies are morally controversial and that the will of the majority may not be morally right. Conscience clauses vary considerably by the object of their concern (i.e., individuals, institutions, or health maintenance or insurance organizations) and the actions they encompass (provision, participation, referral, or payment for services), and while they are not constitutionally required under the free exercise clause of the First Amendment, neither are they forbidden by its establishment clause.[56]

Because the maintenance of public order requires the placement of limits on the exercise of conscience, societies must determine how and where conscientious objection should be allowed. One justification for restricting liberty of conscience is based on liberty itself. Rawls takes this view, claiming that our shared interest in public order leads to the recognition that social stability is a necessary condition for our life pursuits, including the fulfillment of our own moral and religious obligations.[57] Therefore, says Rawls, governments should impartially constrain liberty of conscience only when to do otherwise would be expected to result in significant damage to public order, security, or welfare. The challenge lies in determining what threats to society justify constraints on conscience, and this inevitably requires weighing one freedom against another.

As federal legislation increases access to health care and imposes additional service obligations on health care providers, the balance of legal protections might be expected to shift toward patient access, unless protections for conscientious practice by clinicians are sustained and strengthened. The perceived need for more federal protection can be seen in the Respect for Rights of Conscience Act of 2011, proposed as an amendment to the Patient Protection and Affordable Care Act (PPACA) passed by the U.S. Congress in 2010. This amendment, which has not yet been passed, includes broad protections for health care providers, stipulating that nothing in PPACA "shall be construed to require an individual or institutional health care provider, or authorize a health plan to require a provider, to provide, participate in, or refer for a specific item or service contrary to the provider's religious beliefs or moral convictions" and that "a health plan shall not be considered to have failed to provide timely or other access to items or services under this title (or any amendment made by this title) or to fulfill any other requirement

[56] White, "Crisis of conscience."

[57] Rawls, *A theory of justice*, 211–15.

under this title because it has respected the rights of conscience of such a provider pursuant to this paragraph."[58]

Conscience clauses serve an immediate practical function for individual professionals and institutions who find themselves caught in conflicts between professional conscience and patient preference. They also represent a society's acknowledgment of the deeply controversial nature of some medical services and its commitment to honor liberty of conscience by allowing individual professionals to practice in ways consistent with their deepest moral convictions. As such, conscience clauses are highly significant, both as legal provisions protecting the liberty rights of professionals and as social indicators of irreconcilable differences within a morally pluralistic society.

Without denying this significance, we should note that conscience clauses have their limitations. For instance, they can be crafted so narrowly as to provide little in the way of actual legal protection, especially when they address institutions rather than individuals. For example, a Catholic hospital may not be considered religious enough to satisfy the qualifying requirements of a statutory conscience clause because it does not care for the sick for distinctively religious purposes or does not serve only Catholics.[59] Conscience clauses may also be faulted for not covering enough types of health care providers or kinds of procedures or services and because they are sometimes circumvented, associated with ineffective remedies, or given unsympathetic interpretations by courts.[60] Finally, there may be employment practices that have the potential to make conscience clauses practically useless by discriminating against professionals with conscientious objections.[61]

Another potential limitation to conscience clauses concerns the scope of their application, that is, whether they should apply to individuals *and* institutions. Some maintain that hospitals, clinics, and other health care institutions should not be given the same liberties as individuals. They claim that the right of personal or spiritual conscience is not available to a hospital corporation, "which may have an artificial legal personality but not a spiritual personality protected by human rights laws,"[62] or that health care facilities "lack a moral being and consequently cannot

[58] H.R. 1179: Respect for Rights of Conscience Act of 2011.
[59] Pellegrino, "The physician's conscience, conscience clauses, and religious belief."
[60] Wardle, "Protecting the rights of conscience of health care providers."
[61] R. Walley, "A question of conscience," *British Medical Journal* 1 (1976): 1456–58.
[62] Dickens and Cook, "The scope and limits of conscientious objection."

suffer metaphysical consequences for their choices."[63] By contrast, others believe that there is such a thing as "institutional conscience" that should be respected, because institutions are collections of individuals devoted to a shared organizational mission and set of ethical principles.[64] On this view, an institution functions like a moral agent, based on the decisions its leaders make and for which they are morally accountable. Seen this way, an institution can be said to have a conscience,[65] a notion that harmonizes with society's support for the organization of legal entities to achieve purposes best accomplished by collective action. In health care, these purposes represent moral values and ends, such as healing, comforting, and curing. In support of institutional conscience, Lynn Wardle observes that society makes laws that "recognize the entities created for such moral purposes, considers them legal 'persons,' and extends significant legal benefits to them (including tax exemptions, immunity from liability, and the like) when they advance certain moral goals favored by the state."[66] It is a mistake, he argues, to draw a line between individuals and institutions, since institutions are simply collections of individuals acting in association with each other to accomplish moral ends to which these individuals are committed.

A final area of concern involves the distinction between public and private enterprises. Some argue that when an institution exists as a publicly supported or governed entity, or a professional serves in a publicly supported or governed role, patients should be able to receive legal medical services from a professional working in such an entity or serving in such a role without any limitations imposed by conscience clauses. This appears to be the position Katherine White takes by suggesting that when a health professional is defined as a "state actor," she should have to yield her conscientious concerns so that patients can have access to care that would otherwise be available save for those concerns.[67] Martha Minow similarly maintains that a physician who works at a publicly supported hospital is differently situated (than a professional functioning as a private individual) in a way that is morally and legally relevant, and this difference ought to constrain the extent to which such a physician's liberty of conscience should be allowed to limit patients' access to care. She also doubts the validity of the private–public distinction given the role that public

[63] Wilson, "The limits of conscience."
[64] Pellegrino, "The physician's conscience, conscience clauses, and religious belief."
[65] Sulmasy, "What is conscience and why is respect for it so important?"
[66] Wardle, "Protecting the rights of conscience of health care providers."
[67] White, "Crisis of conscience."

monies play in so much of the delivery and funding of health care.[68] In contrast to White and Minow, Wardle focuses on the conflict of values in the government's desire to provide efficient access to controversial medical services while simultaneously wanting to protect the rights of conscience of health professionals. He believes that the best approach to this conflict is to allow one value to take precedence over another and holds that rights of conscientious refusal have the stronger claim. The conflict, he argues, cannot be solved by drawing a private–public distinction because conscience transcends such distinctions: individuals working in public domains are no less entitled to protections of conscience than those working in private domains.[69]

With the introduction of mandated contraception coverage under the Patient Protection and Affordable Care Act in 2010, there has been an escalation in the public debate over institutional conscience. The issue involves the extent to which legal accommodations should be available to protect the institutional conscience of religious organizations, including hospitals that provide health insurance plans for their employees and have religious or moral objections to contraception, sterilization, and abortion-inducing drugs.[70] Some argue that the government has a compelling interest in ensuring that contraceptive coverage is provided to women and that requiring this coverage does not violate employers' rights to the free exercise of religion.[71] Others disagree, arguing that the new law is an assault on religious liberty and the rights of conscience and that the government oversteps its bounds by taking upon itself the prerogative of determining what qualifies as a religious ministry by allowing some religious organizations (e.g., churches) to be exempt from providing such insurance plans, but not others (e.g., religiously affiliated hospitals or schools).[72] The depth of concern for religious freedom in this matter has resulted in numerous lawsuits from well-known institutions and given rise to the impression among some observers that this disagreement

68 Minow, "On being a religious professional."

69 Wardle, "Protecting the rights of conscience of health care providers."

70 Matthew C. Harrison and Samuel Rodriguez, "HHS mandate: an attack on all people of faith," *Washington Post*, August 9, 2012.

71 Destyn D. Stallings, "A tough pill to swallow: whether the Patient Protection and Affordable Care Act obligates Catholic organizations to cover their employees' prescription contraceptives," *Tulsa Law Review* 48 (2012): 117–41.

72 John Garvey et al., "Unacceptable," www.becketfund.org/wp-content/uploads/2012/04/Unacceptable-4-11.pdf.

represents a historic confrontation in the United States between church and state.[73]

IV. SHOULD THE LEGITIMACY OF CONSCIENTIOUS OBJECTION DEPEND ON CLINICAL CONTEXT?

When evaluating the extent to which conscience is respected within the medical profession, it is important that we ask whether assessments of the legitimacy of conscience may depend on clinical context. For instance, what if conscientious objection to participation in decisions intending to end life in utero (i.e., abortion) is less likely to be taken seriously than conscientious objection to participation in decisions intending to prolong life in the intensive care unit when the likelihood of survival is very small or the so-called quality of life is very poor (i.e., the problem of medical futility)? If we find that assessments of the legitimacy of conscientious objection vary from context to context – that is, if the legitimacy of conscience is treated as if it were context-dependent – then it may be appropriate to conclude that something more than conscience is at issue in these assessments.

One possibility is that primary ethical judgments about features specific to different clinical contexts determine the perceived legitimacy of conscience in those contexts, rather than primary assessments of conscience itself. On this view, clinical contexts perceived by professional organizations, committees, or commentators as morally unacceptable or controversial will lead to more positive assessments of conscientious objection; by contrast, clinical contexts perceived as morally acceptable or uncontroversial will lead to more negative assessments of conscientious objection. Such a dependence – if it exists – need not be viewed as duplicitous or conniving, for when we view moral reasoning as a basic dimension of conscience, we should not be surprised to find an association between primary ethical judgments about features specific to clinical contexts (e.g., the morality of abortion or medical futility) and claims of conscience related to those contexts. It may well be the case that at least some assessments of the legitimacy of conscientious objection in a given clinical context are surrogate markers for ethical judgments about that clinical context. I am inclined to think that this is, in fact, the case.

[73] L. Martin Nussbaum, "Church v. state: the historic lawsuits over the HHS abortifacient/contraceptive mandate," November 15, 2012, www.preservereligiousfreedom.org/2012/11/church-v-state-the-historic-lawsuits-over-the-hhs-abortifacientcontraceptive-mandate/.

On the basis of the following selective review of assessments of conscientious objection within different clinical contexts, it is clear that conscience (or conscientious objection) evokes a wide range of responses from its commentators: *concern* about harms that may flow from freedom of conscience; *appreciation* for the moral struggle and tension conscientious objection represents; *respect* for professional prerogative and moral freedom; *admiration* for courageous action inspired by conscience; and *unqualified support* when, as integrity, it is viewed as an essential ingredient of professionalism. It seems that conscience is alternately admired and questioned, depending on the context, and this variability presses the question of whether sometimes there is something other than the "substance" of conscience that is driving the assessment of its worth.

A. Human Reproduction

In the clinical context of human reproduction (i.e., abortion, contraception, and sterilization), advocates of patient autonomy place moral priority on the patient's "right to hold certain views, make certain choices, and take certain actions based on personal values and beliefs"[74] and describe respect for professional conscience as "one of many values"[75] that should be "reasonably accommodated" only when patients' "rights to medically indicated and lawful care are not compromised."[76] Such assessments portray professional conscience as a potential impediment or threat to patient autonomy and, as such, as a matter of significant moral concern.

B. Physician-Assisted Suicide

In the context of legalized physician-assisted suicide, discussion of conscience may include a respectful recognition of the moral tension that arises when a clinician is at moral odds with his patient, profession, or society. For example, a hospice professional in a state in which physician-assisted suicide is legal might be opposed to this practice because of its emphasis on self-deliverance and its contradiction of the traditional moral vision of hospice of enhancing quality of life without intending to end life. The tension between the comfort-oriented purposes of hospice and the

74 ACOG, "The limits of conscientious refusal in reproductive medicine."
75 Ibid.
76 Dickens and Cook, "The scope and limits of conscientious objection."

death-facilitating purposes of physician-assisted suicide can create intense pressures on professionals who practice where assisted suicide has been legalized, because their moral integrity prevents them from assisting efforts to end life intentionally.[77] The hospice community is respectfully aware of the need to honor this tension, especially since there is opposition to physician-assisted suicide at the organizational level.[78] The perceived legitimacy of conscientious objection to assisted suicide is also evidenced by conscience clauses in state statutes protecting the professional right to avoid participation in assisted suicide.

C. Medical Futility

The issue of medical futility has in recent years attracted significant attention from clinicians, professional societies, hospitals (some of which have developed futility policies), and even states. A Texas law provides the steps physicians must take when refusing to follow the life-sustaining treatment preferences of patients or families when those preferences are deemed medically unreasonable. The breadth and depth of professional opposition to treatments deemed futile represent a remarkable display of professional autonomy in an era of medicine that is otherwise habitually focused on respecting patient autonomy. The professional push against futile treatment is premised on the professional's ability – some would say responsibility – to determine when medical treatments are futile and on the professional's prerogative to discontinue treatments when such a determination has been made or to disengage from patients if futile treatments are continued. Whether or not conscience is explicitly invoked, futility policies imply a right of conscience because they assume that physicians, or hospitals, should not be forced to provide medical treatments that professionals believe run contrary to their best medical and ethical judgments – that is, contrary to their beliefs and values. This assumption is held so firmly that it is taken as a justification for unilateral decisions that contradict the wishes of patients and families. Futility policies show how ready some physicians and institutions are to contravene a patient's or family's wishes when they believe that a patient or family is wrong.

77 Courtney S. Campbell, Jan Hare, and Pam Matthews, "Conflicts of conscience: hospice and assisted suicide," *Hastings Center Report* 25, no. 3 (1995): 36–43.

78 "Commentary and Resolution on Physician Assisted Suicide" (National Hospice & Palliative Care Organization, 2005).

To illustrate this readiness, consider the following examples. The AMA's policy on futile care declares that patients "should not be given treatments simply because they demand them,"[79] and though its policy on medical futility in end-of-life care supports due process to resolve conflicts, it reserves the right – when conflicts are intractable – for transfer to another physician or another institution or, if neither is feasible, refusal to offer a desired treatment.[80] The ACOG likewise maintains, in its general position statement on medical futility, that although "the values of the patient and the preservation of life ordinarily take priority," when conflicts over futility are insoluble and transfer to another physician or facility is not feasible, "caregivers are not required to provide care that they regard as medically futile."[81] The ACOG also addresses futility in position statements specific to end-of-life care. In a 1995 statement, the ACOG held that a physician "cannot be compelled to violate personal ethical or religious commitments in the service of the patient's good" and "is not obliged to do something that is at odds with his or her conscience."[82] A revision of this statement in 2008 continues to insist that "a patient's demand for care that she deems desirable is not sufficient to impose on providers an absolute obligation to provide care that is futile or likely to be harmful without offering corresponding benefit."[83] But the 2008 revision differs from the 1995 statement in important ways: it qualifies the categorical nature of its opposition to any violation of the physician's individual commitments (stating that physicians "*usually* cannot be compelled to violate personal ethical or religious commitments"; emphasis added), and it omits any mention of conscience and the impropriety of acting against it. This notable shift in language from 1995 to 2008 is unexplained. As one last example from a major professional organization, the AAP states that physicians "generally can refuse to perform actions that they consider medically inappropriate," such as prescribing antibiotics for a viral infection or performing surgery that has an

[79] AMA, Code of Medical Ethics, "Opinion 2.035: futile care" (1994); www.ama-assn.org/ama/pub/physician-resources/medical-ethics/code-medical-ethics/opinion2035.page.

[80] AMA, Code of Medical Ethics, "Opinion 2.037: medical futility in end-of-life care" (1997); www.ama-assn.org/ama/pub/physician-resources/medical-ethics/code-medical-ethics/opinion2037.page.

[81] ACOG, Committee on Ethics, "Medical futility (ACOG committee opinion no. 362)," *Obstetrics and Gynecology* 109 (2007): 791–94.

[82] ACOG, Committee on Ethics, "End-of-life decision making: understanding goals of care," *International Journal of Gynecology & Obstetrics* 50 (1995): 208–14.

[83] ACOG, Committee on Ethics, "End-of-life decision making (committee report no. 403)," *Obstetrics and Gynecology* 111 (2008): 1021–27.

unacceptably high mortality rate,[84] noting that such refusals are based on medical knowledge, not on moral, religious, or political beliefs, and are therefore not like conscientious objections.

These examples from the AMA, the ACOG, and the AAP show how the professional response to medical futility has been framed largely as a matter of medical expertise that validates the prerogative of professionals to make medical judgments that take precedence over patient or family preferences. The professional response to medical futility represents a departure from what can otherwise be seen as a habitual deference to patient autonomy in contemporary medicine. It is also worth noting that discussions of medical futility sometimes assume that futility judgments are a matter of medical knowledge and expertise, not moral evaluation (witness the AAP statement). As intuitive as such assumptions can be for physicians, the discussion in Chapter 1 about the inseparability between clinical decisions and ethical values endeavors to demonstrate that any attempt to separate the "medical" from the "ethical" aspects of clinical practice are inherently problematic. Though there are clinical circumstances in which medical facts appear to be overwhelmingly dispositive for decision making (e.g., when a patient with metastatic cancer refractory to anti-cancer treatment is in septic shock despite treatment with multiple antibiotics and vasopressor medications), in general we should be willing to question the validity of discussions of medical futility that treat clinical decision making as if medical facts were somehow detachable from ethical beliefs and values associated with those facts.

D. Childhood Vaccinations

Another clinical context in which questions of conscience among professionals can arise involves parents who refuse to allow their children to receive routine childhood vaccinations. Survey data suggest that a substantial proportion of pediatricians dismiss families from their care for refusing vaccinations (39 percent would dismiss a family for refusing all vaccines, and 28 percent would dismiss a family for refusing select vaccines),[85] and the Bioethics Committee of the AAP respects the prerogative of the pediatrician to "encourage the family to find another physician or practice"

[84] AAP, "Policy statement."

[85] Erin A. Flanagan-Klygis, Lisa Sharp, and Joel E. Frader, "Dismissing the family who refuses vaccines: a study of pediatrician attitudes," *Archives of Pediatrics and Adolescent Medicine* 159 (2005): 929–34.

in cases "when a substantial level of distrust develops, significant differences in the philosophy of care emerge, or poor quality of communication persists."[86]

E. Financial Incentives, Organizational Misconduct, and Medical Error Disclosure

The exercise of conscience can evoke admiration when it is associated with courageous professional action on behalf of patients when their interests are threatened by financial expediency or institutional misconduct. For instance, commentators recognize that physicians need integrity to resist organizational and economic pressures that would have physicians become "commercial entrepreneurs, gateclosers, or agents of fiscal policy" that contradict the covenant of trust at the center of the physician–patient relationship.[87] Such resistance may be needed in managed-care settings where noncooperation with financial incentives that cut against patients' interests may require conscientious objection, withdrawal, or even whistleblowing.[88] The willingness to object to organizational misconduct illustrates the need for conscience-driven professionals who serve as guardians of the ethical values that sustain the patient-oriented missions of health care institutions.[89] Medical errors create another clinical context in which conscience can be seen as motivating physicians to do what they believe is right in the midst of highly potent pressures that encourage silence and deception instead of straightforward communication with patients about what has happened.[90]

F. Professionalism and Integrity

Finally, it is common to find unqualified support for integrity in discussions about medical professionalism. A widely affirmed physician charter

[86] Douglas S. Diekema and American Academy of Pediatrics Committee on Bioethics, "Responding to parental refusals of immunization of children," *Pediatrics* 115 (2005): 1428–31.

[87] Crawshaw et al., "Patient–physician covenant."

[88] Childress, "Appeals to conscience."

[89] T. Faunce, S. Bolsin, and W. P. Chan, "Supporting whistleblowers in academic medicine: training and respecting the courage of professional conscience," *Journal of Medical Ethics* 30 (2004): 40–43.

[90] Lauris C. Kaldjian et al., "An empirically derived taxonomy of factors affecting physicians' willingness to disclose medical errors," *Journal of General Internal Medicine* 21 (2006): 942–48.

on professionalism begins with reference to the fundamental need for "the integrity of both individual physicians and the whole profession" if the public's trust in physicians is to be preserved,[91] and integrity is included when the ethical virtues and values of professionalism are enumerated.[92] Granted, integrity is more often mentioned than defined in such discussions, and its relationship to conscience may not be acknowledged. But I would suggest that reference to integrity as a core feature of professionalism should be taken as an invitation to recognize the importance of conscience in the medical professional when both integrity and conscience are understood as requiring, among other things, a basic consistency between what a professional believes and how a professional acts.

The preceding paragraphs illustrate that conscience evokes diverse responses from commentators depending on the clinical context under consideration. This suggests that an assessment of the legitimacy of conscience in a given clinical context may at times be an indicator of a primary ethical judgment (i.e., a conclusion of moral reasoning) about that clinical context rather than a primary assessment of the legitimacy of conscientious objection in and of itself. As suggested earlier, if moral reasoning is an essential element of conscience, we should not be surprised if conscience is invoked by some and questioned by others in the course of moral dialogues and debates about ethical issues that matter deeply to health care professionals.

We will be more likely to have clear discussions (as well as clear disagreements) if we can separate our assessments of the moral significance of conscience from our assessments of the significance of the moral beliefs and values upon which we base our ethical judgments about specific clinical contexts as we discuss their morally relevant details. If engaged carefully, such discussions should reveal an intimate relationship between claims of conscience and conclusions of moral reasoning. But as described in Chapter 5, claims of conscience by themselves should not be taken to be self-justifying. Rather, they should be accompanied by explanations of how moral beliefs and values are related to moral positions or actions, which is a matter of moral reasoning. As an ultimate *subjective* moral norm,

91 ABIM Foundation (American Board of Internal Medicine), "Medical professionalism in the new millennium: a physician charter," *Annals of Internal Medicine* 136 (2002): 243–46.

92 Michael D. Brennan, "Professionalism and academic medicine: the Mayo Clinic program in professionalism," *Irish Journal of Medical Science* 177 (2008): 23–27; Cohen, "Linking professionalism to humanism"; Jack Coulehan, "Today's professionalism: engaging the mind but not the heart," *Academic Medicine* 80 (2005): 892–98; Swick, "Toward a normative definition of medical professionalism."

a claim of conscience will always signal to the listener that the speaker believes she is bound by the conclusion she has reached – for that conclusion represents the final and best assessment of what she believes is right, even if that assessment may in fact be wrong.

V. SHIFTING THE FOCUS FROM CONSCIENTIOUS OBJECTION TO CONSCIENTIOUS PRACTICE

Discussions about conscience in the practice of medicine tend to center on moral disagreements or conflicts in which a professional refuses to participate in an action that he finds morally objectionable. As a result, these discussions are usually categorized as dealing with *conscientious objection* or *conscientious refusal*, thereby emphasizing what can be called the *negative* work of conscience. However, the reasons, feelings, and motivations that constitute conscience – and function to preserve moral integrity by ensuring consistency between moral belief and moral action – not only repel a person away from morally objectionable actions, but also attract a person to morally desirable goals. In this sense, conscience also does what we can call *positive* work. We can place the totality of the impact of conscience – both its positive and negative work – under the more general category of *conscientious practice*.

Given some of the historical interpretations of conscience presented in Chapter 4, it is not too surprising that the potential of conscience to move a person away from objectionable things has received more attention than its potential to move a person toward desirable things. The negative work of conscience is especially visible when conscience is viewed as having an essentially punitive function. In casual conversation we are more likely to hear mention of conscience as something that is active because of a bad deed done and now regretted ("He is suffering from a guilty conscience") than because of a good deed done and now celebrated ("He is enjoying a satisfied conscience"). Such an imbalanced view of conscience is unfortunate and untrue to the many historical and contemporary conceptions that defensibly view conscience not merely as an internal source of self-criticism and guilt, but as a positive moral resource that forms ethical sensibilities, promotes cultivation of the virtues, and motivates action that allows our deepest and most authentic moral commitments to be manifested in how we decide to live.[93]

[93] Langston, *Conscience and other virtues*, 119.

This positive work of conscience, in concert with the virtues, represents an essential moral resource for sustaining the practice of medicine in all its daily but inevitably significant routines. These routines are significant because any contact with a patient is an opportunity to place the needs and dignity of a particular person at the center of a health professional's field of moral vision. Beyond the need to sustain motivation to meet the daily challenges of medical practice, the positive work of conscience is needed to sustain commitment to the internal goods of medicine amid potentially distorting influences that emerge when health care enterprises pursue external goods that may focus inordinately on money, power, and prestige.[94] In extreme cases, for instance, a professional may need to rely on conscience and courage to be a "whistleblower" against institutional corruption[95] or, less dramatically, to resist financial pressures that compromise patients' interests in the setting of managed care.[96] Conscience can be seen as the moral resource for the kind of professionalism that is rigorous enough to motivate advocacy, dissent, and even disobedience or principled exit from an unacceptable work environment.[97] Conscience, along with courage, is also required when health professionals are called to risk their safety, health, or lives during times of disaster.[98]

The overarching significance of the positive work of conscience is displayed when writers encourage us to see the interdependence between a professional's conscience and her basic motivation for service as a health care professional. This interdependence implies that when physicians feel compelled to act against their consciences, they not only compromise their ethical integrity, but also are susceptible to the corrosive effect a compromised conscience can have on the dedication needed to sustain patient care.[99] The interdependence between conscience and service can inspire deep and enduring convictions that establish a moral imperative to care well for patients and criticize practices that run contrary to their interests.[100]

94 MacIntyre, *After virtue*, 194.
95 Faunce, Bolsin, and Chan, "Supporting whistleblowers in academic medicine."
96 Childress, "Conscience and conscientious actions in the context of MCOs."
97 M. K. Wynia et al., "Medical professionalism in society," *New England Journal of Medicine* 341 (1999): 1612–16.
98 AMA, Code of Medical Ethics, "Opinion 9.067: physician obligation in disaster preparedness and response" (2004); www.ama-assn.org/ama/pub/physician-resources/medical-ethics/code-medical-ethics/opinion9067.page.
99 Bleich, "The physician as a conscientious objector."
100 Minow, "On being a religious professional."

Given the physical, emotional, and existential demands that medical practice imposes on physicians, it would be strange, even self-defeating, if the medical profession did not welcome persons into its ranks who have conscience-based motivations that, due to their depth and significance, can be expected to enhance a health professional's ability to meet the challenges health care entails – such as overwork, fatigue, continuous learning, bureaucratic frustrations, conflicts of interest, and the temptation to take advantage of the patient–physician relationship. Whether such motivations are categorized under conscience or integrity, the medical profession would benefit from more candor and discussion about the foundational beliefs and values that students and physicians rely on to sustain an attitude and habit of service to patients. We should also consider how to cultivate and support these motivational resources, especially during the formative years of training. The more clearly we see the role played by conscience in sustaining the work of health professionals, the more likely we will see the foundational beliefs and values it entails as part of the web of moral resources the medical profession needs to sustain its healing mission. Talk about ethics and professionalism will ring hollow if those hearing it lack the motivation to strive for the standards and ideals our health professions celebrate.

The need for deep sources of motivation is perhaps most obvious when a professional must sacrifice something of value in the course of serving those in medical need, such as when a physician or nurse knowingly goes into harm's way to serve the victims of an epidemic or disaster. But these sources are also essential to sustain a patient-centered professional ethos amid the routine and daily pressures of an increasingly regulated and managed practice environment. For instance, commentators are right to wonder how financial incentives, designed to motivate physicians to improve the quality of patient care, may fail to appreciate what really interests physicians. In contrast to a narrow financial focus, it is reasonable to assume that physicians can be expected to be motivated by intrinsic values related to the satisfactions of completing complex and difficult tasks, achieving good clinical outcomes, and working in a context of autonomy, respect, and meaningful relationships.[101] We can take such reflections about professional values a step further by wondering about the moral motivations that underlie these professional values and galvanize them against the potentially deprofessionalizing effects, for example,

[101] Christine K. Cassel and Sachin H. Jain, "Assessing individual physician performance: does measurement suppress motivation?" *JAMA* 307, no. 24 (2012): 2595–96.

of administrative strategies that replace appeals to patient welfare with appeals to financial self-interest. To acknowledge the contribution that foundational beliefs and values make in the lives of health professionals is to recognize that the motivational source of professional ethics resides finally within the integrity of its individual members. And this integrity must be sustained if the health professions are to flourish.

In the Physician's Oath of the World Medical Association's Declaration of Geneva, physicians are called to practice their profession "with conscience and dignity."[102] This plain statement acknowledges the way in which conscience reflects a professional's deepest moral core and constitutes an essential ingredient of the commitment to serve those in medical need. This statement thereby captures the comprehensive and primary nature of conscientious practice. It also serves as a counter to those critics of conscientious objection who speak as if an individual's moral beliefs and values were somehow secondary to their professional concerns and could be circumvented to avoid interfering with patient care.[103] When the moral beliefs and values of which conscience is composed are recognized as primary and integral to a professional's commitment to medicine, nursing, or pharmacy, it becomes clear that we cannot ignore or sacrifice these beliefs and values without denying the interdependence between conscience and the motivation to serve as a professional. As the World Medical Association's oath indicates, conscience should be seen as a moral resource that ought to pervade professional practice.

VI. WIDER PROFESSIONAL, SOCIAL, AND POLITICAL BENEFITS OF CONSCIENTIOUS PRACTICE

Because questions of conscience tend to focus on individuals and their claims to moral freedom, there may be a tendency to view protections of conscience as societal concessions that benefit only the individuals whose consciences are at issue. Though understandable, such a view fails to appreciate the wider benefits that can flow to the health professions and to society when respect for the freedom of conscience is adequately established in the standards of the health professions and the policies of governments.

102 "Physician's Oath, Declaration of Geneva" (World Medical Association); www.wma.net/en/30publications/10policies/g1/.

103 Cantor and Baum, "The limits of conscientious objection."

For physicians, conscientious practice consists in the ability to practice medicine in a way that is in harmony with one's foundational beliefs and values. The need to explain conscientious practice – for instance, in the setting of a moral disagreement or conflict – involves giving sincere moral reasons for or against certain practices or policies. The reasons provided by the conscientious practitioner will inevitably raise questions about the status quo represented by the authority of administrators, elected officials, or the majority position in an organization or a society. The conscientious practitioner's act of questioning should therefore be expected to prompt institutions, professional organizations, and governments to consider how a given practice or policy may involve uncertainties or controversies about the goals of medicine, the extent of patient and professional responsibilities, the extent of patient and professional freedoms, and need for order in a democratic society. Responses to these areas of concern will necessarily involve assumptions about what is believed to be ultimately real and good, that is, questions about the foundational beliefs and values that support our moral judgments. This kind of questioning should promote debate that clarifies the moral meaning of professional practices. When moral reasoning permeates a professional or civic community, all parties to a disagreement are compelled to sharpen their arguments, refine their best attempts at rational persuasion, and recognize that neither medical science nor governmental policy is self-validating.[104] The exercise of individual conscience prods those in authority to elaborate their reasoning, reminding us that one of the vital functions of conscientious dissent is not to undermine professional or public consensus, but to clarify it.[105] And in extreme situations of moral conflict, freedom of conscience can provide the individual a moral authority that is potent enough to oppose even the most threatening of governments,[106] whether or not opposition proves successful.

The moral reasoning and dialogue inspired by conscientious practice should help us see that philosophical and religious diversity – though it can be the cause of disquieting conflicts – can also be a source of critical appraisal that fuels constructive and vital political debate.[107] The greater

[104] Jean Bethke Elshtain, "Why science cannot stand alone," *Theoretical Medicine and Bioethics* 29 (2008): 161–69.

[105] John H. Hallowell, "Conscience and civil authority," in *Conscience: its freedom and limitations*, ed. William C. Bier (New York: Fordham University Press, 1971), 159–69.

[106] Reinhold Niebuhr, *The children of light and the children of darkness* (New York: Scribner's, 1960), 80–84.

[107] Minow, "On being a religious professional."

the constraint on freedom of conscience in the practice of medicine, the less diversity, debate, and opportunity there will be for democratic processes to identify solutions that are responsive to the needs and interests of *all* patients, professionals, and citizens. Indeed, it is worth wondering what adverse professional and social outcomes are possible when professional or government control in controversial matters results in a sameness of practice that stifles further thinking about such practices.[108] We should note the parallel between freedom of conscience and freedom of speech, with respect to the way both can facilitate social processes that bring us closer to the truth about a given matter.[109]

As great as the professional and social benefits of conscientious practice arguably are, there remains a sense in which the value of conscience is ultimately attributable to individual persons. Respect for conscience is expressed by a society's willingness to honor individual freedom by protecting those aspects of human life that are considered most valuable and may be most vulnerable. According to Martha Nussbaum, governments should protect expression of conscience and religion because both are concerned with questions of ultimate meaning – questions of life and death, ethical foundations, and human fulfillment – and this protection, she maintains, should be limited only when the pursuit of ultimate meaning violates the rights of others or conflicts with some compelling state interest.[110] Nussbaum believes that the importance of this protection is represented in the First Amendment, even though the framers of the Constitution chose to articulate it in terms of religion rather than conscience. For Nussbaum, the First Amendment's free exercise clause reflects the "ideas of equal respect for all citizens' consciences, 'delicate' accommodation of conscientious scruples, and fairness to minorities who live in a majority world."[111]

The foundational beliefs and values that shape a person's conscience are as deep as they are diverse, and persons do not abandon these beliefs and values when they become professionals. As a result, professionals' views on matters such as truth telling, altruism, suicide, and human dignity depend on individual beliefs and values that likely precede their professional training. As Robert Veatch observes, the pre-professional philosophical or religious worldviews that comprise these beliefs and values should

[108] Walley, "A question of conscience."
[109] Granrose, "The authority of conscience," 232.
[110] Nussbaum, *Liberty of conscience*, 168–69.
[111] Ibid., 174.

not be presumed to yield to, or be trumped by, professional sources of ethical norms.[112] The moral reality is that health care professionals – and patients too, of course – ultimately have to decide for themselves which moral beliefs, values, and traditions are authoritative for them. This decision can be understood as a matter of individual conscience, and its outcome will greatly influence what each professional believes the practice of medicine should be.

VII. SUMMARY

It can be difficult to manage tensions that arise when physicians or other health care professionals conscientiously refuse to provide, or facilitate the provision of, certain legally available services because of moral objections. Those who question the validity of such refusals may interpret a professional's unwillingness as a violation of patient autonomy and a failure to fulfill a fiduciary or social obligation. Efforts to manage conscientious refusals usually necessitate balancing the interests of patients (for services), society (for the availability of services), and physicians (for the preservation of integrity). These efforts are reflected in recommendations for disclosure (by giving prior notice, describing alternatives, and explaining the reasons for refusal), facilitation of treatment (by referring or transferring care to another health care professional), provision of treatment (in cases of emergency or when other means of treatment are unavailable), or avoidance of professional work that includes objectionable activities.

Standards of assessment for managing conflicts arising from conscientious objection can be considered according to the way different values are prioritized. A *physician-regulating standard* places first priority on a patient's right to request and receive medical services that are legal and available. A *physician-respecting standard* acknowledges the physician's prima facie obligation to respect and promote patients' treatment preferences while also acknowledging the need to respect and protect the professional's conscience in controversial matters. Both standards respect the right of self-determination of patients, but when conflicts of conscience arise, the physician-regulating standard favors the satisfaction of patient preferences, and the physician-respecting standard favors the protection of professional integrity. The physician-respecting standard presumes a mutual respect for autonomy and conscience between patients and physicians and is compatible with the imposition of serious – but not

[112] Veatch, "The sources of professional ethics."

limitless – unilateral obligations on physicians in light of the asymmetric responsibilities within the patient–physician relationship. Federal and state laws known as conscience clauses reflect this mutual respect by protecting the right of health care professionals and health care institutions to avoid participation in practices to which they object on moral or religious grounds. These laws publicly acknowledge the controversial nature of some medical services, and they reflect the common belief that conscience represents a unique and vital human characteristic that warrants government protection in a morally pluralistic society.

A review of different clinical contexts in which conscientious objection tends to arise suggests that assessments of conscience are not only variable but also context-dependent – implying that something more than conscience is at issue in these assessments. One explanation for this variability is that assessments of the legitimacy of conscientious objection may at times be indicators of a primary ethical judgment (i.e., a conclusion of moral reasoning) about a given clinical context rather than a primary assessment of the legitimacy of conscience itself. In clinical contexts perceived by commentators as morally unacceptable or controversial, assessments of the legitimacy of conscientious objection are likely to be more positive; in those contexts perceived as morally acceptable or uncontroversial, assessments of conscience are likely to be more negative. This context dependency is not surprising. Since moral reasoning should be an essential element of conscience, assessments of the validity of references to conscience in a given context should depend on ethical judgments about that context. However, for increased clarity in our deliberations, we should try to distinguish our assessments of the moral significance of conscience in general from our ethical judgments about specific clinical contexts in particular. For the sake of candor and dialogue, claims of conscience should be accompanied by moral reasoning that explains how moral beliefs and values relate to moral positions or actions. And it is important to remember that when a claim of conscience is made, the person making it is sending a signal to his listeners that he believes he is bound by the moral conclusion he has reached, since conscience is a person's ultimate, albeit subjective, moral norm.

Discussions about conscience in the practice of medicine frequently focus on its negative work (describing things someone is *not* willing to do), and such discussions therefore come under the category of *conscientious objection.* However, the reasons, feelings, and motivations that constitute conscience not only repel individuals away from morally objectionable actions, but also attract them toward morally desirable goals. Conscience therefore also does positive work, and we can place the totality of its impact under the more general category of *conscientious practice*. The positive work of conscience serves as a moral resource that pervades the entire work of a health care professional – forming ethical sensibilities, cultivating virtues, and motivating action. From the influence it has on responses to the daily needs of patients, to moments of exceptional courage and altruism, conscience in the health professions is of overarching significance for the motivation that drives professional service. Given the physical, emotional, and existential demands of medical practice, we do well to acknowledge and support the conscience-based motivations health professionals rely on to meet the challenges health care entails – the work hours, fatigue, bureaucratic frustrations, conflicts of interest, and temptation to take advantage of the patient–physician relationship. The more clearly we see the role played by conscience and the foundational beliefs and values it entails, the more likely we will recognize it as a vital moral resource to help sustain the healing mission of health care.

The pervasive moral significance of conscience explains the difficulty encountered by those who recommend placing certain limits on the free exercise of a medical professional's conscience. Deliberation about such limits will always prove challenging, given the need to balance competing interests and goods in a morally pluralistic society. One of the goods that should be remembered amid these challenges is the social value of questioning and debate. The reasoning that a conscientious practitioner communicates will inevitably raise questions about the status quo and the moral basis of the positions of administrators, majorities, or legislators. Moral reasoning prompts questions that cause institutions, organizations, and governments to consider how practices or policies may include uncertainties or controversies about the goals of medicine, the extent of patient and professional responsibilities, the extent of patient and professional freedoms, and need for order in a democratic society. Reasoned debate sharpens argument and clarifies the nature and extent of consensus. The less freedom of conscience allowed in the practice of medicine, the less diversity, debate, and opportunity there will be to allow democratic processes to identify solutions that are responsive to the needs and interests of *all* patients, professionals, and citizens. But as great as the professional and social benefits of conscientious practice are, its value is ultimately attributable to individual persons. Respect for conscience reveals a society's willingness to protect the expression of what are arguably the most valuable, albeit intangible, aspects of an individual human life – the foundational beliefs and values that define a person's sense of ultimate meaning.

10

An Integrity-Centered Framework for Practical Wisdom in Medicine

In this final chapter I draw from the previous chapters to propose an integrated framework for practical wisdom in medicine, address ways it can be fostered, and then elaborate on some of its implications through four clinical illustrations. The proposed framework depends on ancient and modern insights about elements of practical wisdom, values that ground medicine as a moral practice, responsibilities that guide professional decision making, and the central role that moral integrity ought to play in the life of each medical professional. It is a framework that incorporates goals of care, complementary approaches to normative ethics, conscientious practice, and social obligation – and does so with an awareness of the moral pluralism that exists within the medical profession and society. As envisioned in this framework, practical wisdom involves professional responsiveness to three ethical priorities – the patient, the professional, and society – a responsiveness that requires the integration of values and interests that are usually overlapping but may at times be competing. To successfully accomplish this integration, or at least to do one's best in trying, is an essential part of what it means to have moral integrity in medicine. Virtue ethics provides the inspiration and rationale for this integrity-centered account of professional ethics, one that places a high premium on the moral identity of medical professionals that is inclusive of their fiduciary obligations to patients and accompanying obligations to society.

This framework reflects an essential interdependence between practical wisdom, conscience, and goals of care. It also reflects the conviction that integrity is a requirement for human moral agency and the sustenance of our moral identities as we try to live according to our foundational beliefs and values, reconcile the pursuit of diverse goods, and respond to potentially competing obligations to patients, ourselves, and society. Cultivating the kind of practical wisdom in medicine that this framework recommends is a considerable task, one that requires clear communication about goals of care, ethical reasoning, and background moral beliefs, some of which may reveal sharp disagreements within the morally pluralistic settings of the health professions and society. This cultivation also requires moral imagination and humility, and it invites us to take the formation of conscience or integrity seriously. Within educational environments, practical wisdom can be promoted through instruction and habit-forming practice within a community of professionals committed to common goals and ethical values. Moral diversity among professionals and patients makes for challenges when values conflict and competing interests are hard to reconcile, pointing to the need for a culture of deliberation in which conscientiously held differences are respectfully articulated and engaged. The social contract between professionals and society requires ongoing assessments of the extent to which deep moral differences should be accommodated within the health professions, and that contract should recognize the historically weighty reasons for believing that professionals, patients, and society benefit when conscientious practice is allowed to flourish.

I. A FRAMEWORK FOR PRACTICAL WISDOM IN MEDICINE

Within the tradition of virtue ethics tracing back to Aristotle and Aquinas, practical wisdom (in Greek, *phronesis*; in Latin, *prudentia*) is the foremost of the cardinal virtues because it shows us how to respond realistically – in the sense of being true to reality – when faced with a decision. It is the preeminent practical virtue because a proper understanding of when and how other virtues are to be expressed depends not only on good intentions or desires, but also on the ability to perceive and respond appropriately to the objective features of a situation and the moral values relevant to it. In short, practical wisdom involves the ability to know, and deliberate about, what ends (or goals) are worth pursuing and what means are most likely to accomplish them, and it includes the will to act on the judgments that are reached through deliberation.

As described in Chapter 3, a virtue-based understanding of practical wisdom has five core elements:

1. the pursuit of worthwhile ends (goals) derived from a concept of human flourishing;

2. an accurate perception of the concrete circumstances of a specific practical situation;
3. a commitment to moral virtues and principles that are interdependent and form an integrated moral framework;
4. deliberation that integrates ends (goals), concrete circumstances, and moral virtues and principles; and
5 the motivation to act in order to implement the conclusions reached by such deliberation.

The similarity between practical wisdom and clinical judgment in medicine should be clear, and it can be argued that clinical judgment is, in substance and effect, practical wisdom in the context of medicine. For at its heart, clinical judgment is a matter of looking at (one clinical part of) the world truthfully and then deciding how best to respond to it on the basis of an assessment of the goals to be pursued, the means best suited to achieve those goals, and an appreciation of the moral considerations necessary to guide and motivate medical decision making. Clinical judgment manifests as practical wisdom when ethical purposes, values, and motivations are actively integrated and coherent in clinical decision making. Understanding clinical judgment as practical wisdom reminds us that clinical decision making should always be a moral process because it has to address patients as persons, not merely as biomedical organisms.

The five core elements of practical wisdom in medicine just listed can be summarized by the following five paired concepts:

1. goals of medicine and goals of care;
2. perception and information;
3. principles and virtues;
4. reasoning and integrity; and
5. motivation and action.

These elements form a trajectory of moral decision making that is drawn forward by goals, informed by empirical facts and attributed values, guided by normative principles and virtues, organized through moral reasoning, centered by integrity, and motivated by a desire to make actions consistent with beliefs. I will recapitulate each of these five elements by drawing together facets of discussions from previous chapters in order to place them in this framework of practical wisdom in medicine.

A. Goals of Medicine and Goals of Care

Practical wisdom requires having in view an end (in Greek, *telos*), whether an ultimate end (some form of human flourishing) or an intermediate one (such as health). Goals in health care serve as intermediate ends by providing health care professionals their purpose for action, the basis for assessing the success or failure of action, and grounds for deciding that one possible means to a desired end is better than another. It is helpful to distinguish between *goals of medicine* in general and *goals of care* for specific patients. A group of scholars convened by the Hastings Center drafted a useful list of goals of medicine that they summarized in four domains:

- prevention of disease and injury and promotion and maintenance of health;
- relief of pain and suffering caused by maladies;
- care and cure of those with a malady, and care of those who cannot be cured;
- avoidance of premature death and pursuit of a peaceful death.[1]

Though these goals are familiar, they nevertheless serve as important (albeit general) reference points in policy discussions about the kinds of medical care that should be made available in society.

Goals of care focus on clinical decision making for particular patients and can be listed as follows:

- to cure a patient;
- to help a patient live longer;
- to improve or maintain a patient's function/quality of life/independence;
- to help a patient be comfortable;
- to help a patient achieve his or her life goals;
- to provide support for a patient's family/caregiver; and
- to clarify a patient's diagnosis or prognosis.[2]

Discussing and prioritizing goals of care help patients, families, and clinicians articulate goal-oriented assessments and preferences that can guide shared decision making and increase the likelihood that treatments will be in harmony with patients' values and the reality of their medical

[1] Hanson and Callahan, *The goals of medicine*, 20–30.

[2] Kaldjian et al., "Goals of care toward the end of life"; Haberle et al., "Goals of care among hospitalized patients."

conditions. Once clarified, goals of care allow all those involved to discuss whether a possible intervention makes sense by posing the question, "Will this possible treatment help achieve the agreed-upon goal?" Without agreed-upon goals, medical decisions may be dictated by the urgency of immediate circumstances, access to available treatments, or whatever is considered "usual" care, rather than by the longer-term goals and underlying clinical realities of the patient involved.

The importance of goals of care in decision making shared by patients and professionals is heightened by two features of contemporary medical practice: (1) a tendency among health professionals to view respect for patient autonomy as a matter of eliciting patients' treatment preferences without necessarily discussing the reasons for those preferences and (2) a tendency among health professionals to focus quickly and primarily on interventions rather than first considering the goals those interventions are expected to achieve. Goal-based decision making must, of course, include respect for patient autonomy and discussion of interventional options, but focusing on goals prompts us to go further by engaging in dialogue that situates patient preferences and interventional options against a background of meaning and value that patients can express by describing their goals. By taking a broader and longer view, discussions about goals of care can help counter the tendency to view treatments as somehow self-justifying (i.e., because they are available they are advisable). Goals remind us to ask where we are going before we consider possible ways of getting there.

B. Perception and Information

1. Dimensions of Decision Making: Goals, Probabilities, Suffering, and Cost

In caring for a patient, clinicians need a wide range of knowledge if they are to clearly perceive the patient's world. This knowledge arises from direct interaction with the patient; awareness of her individual psychological, social, and spiritual contexts; the gathering of medical information; training in the diagnosis and treatment of diseases and disorders; and familiarity with the ways that health care can be delivered. Accurate perception of the patient's world includes understanding the patient's goals of care.

But in addition to goals, clinicians need to assess two other key dimensions of the patient's reality that should be incorporated into dialogues that facilitate shared decision making. One of these dimensions focuses on probabilities. Patients need to decide how much value they attribute to different goals of care in light of the statistical probabilities attached to means of achieving those goals. It is not enough to identify and discuss a patient's most important goal of care. A patient also needs to know the likelihood of achieving that goal by means of a given treatment, and a physician needs to know the value a patient attributes to that likelihood. Understanding and discussing probabilities are very challenging in clinical medicine, but whether they are welcome or not, medical practice is guided by an ever-flowing stream of probabilities that are an integral part of evidence-based practice. Even though an individual patient is always a unique case with an uncertain future – rather than an average case with a statistically average future – probabilities rightly matter to clinicians and patients and may sometimes prove decisive in determining whether a treatment is attempted or a goal is pursued.

Another key dimension of the patient's reality that should be incorporated into shared decision making pertains to the patient's willingness to endure suffering and bear the burdens of treatment – whether from physical or emotional pain, disability, dysfunction, social dislocation, rehabilitation, or financial or other hardships that come with the pursuit of medical care. A patient may understand his diagnosis and prognosis, identify his most important goal of care, and accept a given probability of achieving that goal by means of a specific treatment. But there is yet the question of whether he is willing to endure the suffering that may predictably be associated with the treatment considered the most promising means to achieve his goal in his particular circumstances. An otherwise promising treatment may impose such a heavy burden that a patient is unwilling to accept it. Taking these three key dimensions together, clinicians can gain a realistic perception of their patients as persons by knowing their personal, social, and medical details, their goals of care, the value they attribute to outcome probabilities, and their willingness to bear the burdens that treatment requires.

There is one other dimension of shared decision making that may or may not be considered a direct clinical concern, and that is cost. This dimension relates to the financial burdens experienced by individual patients, but it is perhaps more frequently framed as a cost control challenge for society as a whole. The economic costs of health care are now widely recognized as a serious problem in the United States, and it is for good reasons that clinicians are increasingly being encouraged to practice evidence-based and cost-effective medicine. In light of this problem, some would argue that physicians have a dual responsibility: to care for individual patients, one at a time, and simultaneously control health care costs through bedside rationing of health care. But as urgent as economic needs may be, we should be careful not to place directly on the shoulders of clinicians the responsibility of balancing the medical needs of individual patients against the economic needs of society. Given the moral limitations physicians face as human beings in their ability to distribute health care services without favoring some patients and discriminating against others, it would not be realistic to expect them to shoulder the responsibility of micro-allocating resources fairly.

Though cost-controlling decisions in health care are needed, they should be made and implemented through democratic processes of deliberation, policy development, and administrative procedure that allow for a division of labor between those responsible for fair allocation procedures and those responsible for direct patient care. If clinicians are asked to serve simultaneously as advocates for individual patients and as stewards of society's resources, they will be placed in an untenable position. It is challenging enough for physicians to practice medicine according to a professional standard that is patient-centered, evidence-based, and cost-effective, without adding the expectation that they attempt to merge a patient-centered professional standard with a society-centered economic one. When it comes to questions of distributive justice and resource allocation, we should be wary of shifts away from a *primary* focus on the *patient–physician dyad* to what we might call a *patient–physician–population triad.* A division of labor takes *role-fidelity* seriously and helps ensure that individual patients will have advocates in physicians and that populations will have advocates in administrators and legislators.

2. *Directions of Responsibility: Patient, Professional, and Society*

Three landmarks in the wider moral landscape of health care orient the clinician in moral space: the patient, the professional, and society. These landmarks represent three directions of responsibility that have as their moral referents the patient's good, the professional's integrity, and society's needs. They are highly interrelated and can usually be expected to be mutually overlapping and reinforcing. However, there are times when a health care professional will need to navigate tensions that predictably arise within the triangle of responsibilities that joins the professional's integrity with her fiduciary obligations to patients and her professional obligations to society. The resource allocation challenges just discussed are only one example. Because the framework of practical wisdom offered here arises from the person-centered concerns of virtue ethics, it is anchored in the integrity of the individual professional, even as it is interlinked with fundamental commitments to patients and society.

The professional's *responsibility to herself* reflects the irreplaceable and guiding role of this integrity, which can be understood as an imperative to live one's life with the goal of being at unity with oneself. Integrity entails a constellation of moral beliefs, values, commitments, and actions that together constitute not only our choices and purposes, but also our identities. It involves personal wholeness, completeness, and harmony, and it resists compartmentalization as we move from one social context to another. Integrity is the virtue that binds all other virtues and values into a single moral character and links our ethical actions over a lifetime to the ends that guide our individual lives. The integrating function of integrity motivates clinicians to reconcile competing values and goods and to seek practical wisdom in order to navigate tensions that may arise between their conscientious practice and the preferences of patients or the decisions of society.

The professional's *responsibility to the patient* is based on his fiduciary obligation to act in the patient's interests and respect the patient's autonomy as expressed by the patient's values and goals. The fulfillment of this responsibility must incorporate biological and technical realities as understood by medical science, which means that decision making shared by patients and physicians must always have a dual grounding in ethics and science. Patients and physicians bring to the clinical encounter their own personalities, values, beliefs, and motivations that will largely determine how a given patient–physician interaction unfolds, which makes the inseparability of scientific knowledge and ethical value all the more significant. Within the tradition of virtue ethics it is believed that moral character determines how people act; on this view, responsibility to the patient requires physicians to act habitually in the interests of their patients, especially when other, lesser interests compete for the physician's attention.

The professional's *responsibility to society* arises from the "social contract" between society and the medical profession, which comes with mutual obligations and benefits. Central to the contract is the expectation that a physician will fulfill her healing role through altruistic service, respect for patient autonomy, commitment to ethical values, promotion of the public good, and acceptance of appropriately established cost-controlling policies. By entering the medical profession, physicians assume specific commitments that create special professional responsibilities that determine the scope and necessity of their professional service. This necessity is, in one sense, a restriction of a professional's individual freedom; but because it is voluntarily assumed and personally valued, what might otherwise be described as a restriction of individual freedom is more accurately seen as a manifestation of personal commitment to pursue some goods (e.g., a patient's well-being) above others (e.g., a professional's convenience or inordinate financial gain).

But some expectations of society may be perceived by some professionals as inappropriate restrictions when those expectations contradict moral commitments that are of primary importance to the professional. Such expectations engender debate because of disagreements surrounding the relative importance of patient autonomy and professional autonomy, controversies over what should be considered a medical service, and contrasting assessments of the extent to which a professional's freedom of conscience should be honored when moral issues of primary importance are at stake. The inevitable tensions between society's prerogative to impose its will on medicine and the medical professional's prerogative to exercise independent judgment and action call for an ongoing commitment to dialogue and deliberation. Because of moral pluralism, controversial clinical practices, and the enduring value of the freedom of conscience, these tensions will persist.

C. Principles and Virtues

Practical wisdom requires moral grounding so that the ends of decision making, and the means to those ends, are guided and justified by identifiable moral standards that form an overarching moral frame of reference. The framework for practical wisdom offered here assumes a normative ethical grounding in virtue ethics, deontology, and limited consequentialism that is evidenced by a commitment to an interdependent and integrated set of moral virtues and principles. Being integrity-centered, this framework places virtue at the center of normative ethics. This is an acknowledgment of the vital importance of individual moral discernment in social settings that are culturally diverse and morally pluralistic. But this framework also recognizes the contributions of additional sources of ethical value and therefore invites consideration of the relationship between virtues, principles, and consequentialism.

Virtue-based and principle-based ethics enjoy a close and complementary relationship and are best viewed as friends rather than rivals. The correspondence between individual virtues and their corollary principles – for instance, the virtue of *benevolence* and the principle of *beneficence* – shows how seamless the relationships between many virtues and principles can be. As formal prescriptive norms, principles can be seen as having a certain objectivity that is external to the subjectivity of an individual's character. This objectivity can provide rational justification in ethical deliberation. By contrast, virtues can be seen as providing the internal drive and motivation for moral action that principles, as abstract norms, lack. When considering ethical questions from the contrasting vantage points of virtues and principles, we should expect to find a fundamental harmony arising from their complementarity: principles provide direction for moral action, and their corresponding virtues represent character traits that motivate people to act according to the norms that principles prescribe.

Virtue ethics and consequentialism are usually viewed as rivals rather than friends. While virtues and their corollary principles both provide a certain normative stability in ethical decision making, consequentialism provides a certain flexibility that arises from calibrating the moral rightness of particular actions according to the assessed value of predicted outcomes. This flexibility may be perceived as a weakness or a strength. In the practice of medicine, where ethical judgments routinely include assessments of likely outcomes, reasoning based on likely consequences is intuitive, ingrained, and necessary. Predicted outcomes regarding benefits and risks are essential to moral assessments and stand unavoidably alongside principles and virtues. However, it is one thing to take into consideration the anticipated balance of consequences and another to adopt consequentialism formally as a guiding conceptual framework. (Formal approaches to consequentialism tend to adopt a single principle that defines some unidimensional good – such as happiness, preference satisfaction, or financial cost – as the basic measure of right action.) Rejecting too heavy a reliance on consequentialist considerations allows us to avoid two weaknesses of consequentialist theory. First, we avoid pretending that we can predict all potentially relevant future consequences of a given action in the face of the unforeseeable character of human affairs and medical outcomes. Second, we avoid treating all goods and values – such as happiness, years of life, cost, and integrity – as if they were commensurable, that is, capable of comparison on a single scale measurement.

Problems with consequentialism should never keep us from taking consequences seriously, nor should they keep us from considering whether virtue ethics as employed in ethical discussions at times seems to undervalue the importance of outcomes. Moreover, there is a sense in which virtue ethics itself is concerned with consequences because its overarching teleological orientation entails ends that guide the process of moral reasoning, as seen clearly in the way practical wisdom focuses on achieving goals. To the extent that moral action aims at goals, it always takes the consequences of action seriously. Having said this, we must not forget that virtue ethics ascribes a moral significance to virtues that is, in the end, morally independent of consequences.

Taken together, the continuities and contrasts between virtues, principles, and consequences encourage us to adopt a multifaceted approach to ethical reasoning in which these three sources of moral value are coordinated, integrated, and, when certain goods or values are incommensurable, prioritized.

D. Reasoning and Integrity

Moral reasoning that depends on virtues, principles, and consequences is challenged by the moral pluralism of Western societies. This pluralism deprives the health professions of a comprehensive moral consensus that can specify and prioritize relevant virtues, principles, and consequences. We cannot resolve the problem of pluralism by supposing the existence of some morally neutral vantage point. Such a vantage point is unavailable, as the value-loaded practice of medicine makes all too apparent. There is also a sense in which pluralism is reflected in ethics itself, because of the multiple, contrasting values inherent in the moral life (e.g., the value of economic utility vs. the value of individual integrity). These contrasting values lead some persons to conclude that the ethical landscape is inescapably fragmented, and others to hold that though the contrasting goods of the moral life are in tension, they can be given an overarching means of reconciliation and prioritization. On any view, ethical decision making requires moral orientation – some sort of moral compass – whether provided by a developed moral framework or a simple statement of moral priorities. The need for such orientation inevitably raises questions about the foundational beliefs that guide moral reasoning.

Foundational beliefs may be expressed in religious or philosophical terms. Given the debates that surround religious beliefs in Western societies and their scientifically informed communities, it is important to clarify what religious beliefs, as opposed to philosophical ones, should be taken to signify in the context of ethics. If we focus on the function of foundational beliefs in ethical reasoning – the way these beliefs shape our thinking about ethics and its applications – there is no compelling reason to draw a line of separation between religious and philosophical beliefs. The essential point John Reeder makes is that the stereotypical division between religious and nonreligious moral traditions loses its relevance to ethics once it is recognized that all moral perspectives make claims about what is believed to be *good* in light of what is recognized as *real*.[3] On this account, *all* moral frameworks, whether labeled religious or nonreligious, make claims that entail foundational beliefs about what is *ultimately real* and *ultimately good* – beliefs that in turn determine the values, commitments, and actions that characterize ethical decision making. *Foundational beliefs* can therefore be religious or philosophical, so long as they play a foundational role in moral reasoning. Because all moral frameworks make fundamental claims about what is real and good, foundational beliefs are unavoidable in moral reasoning. And because foundational beliefs go all the way down to the roots of our moral frameworks, they will inevitably have practical manifestations.

One of the central concerns of this book is to describe the close relationships among moral reasoning, practical wisdom, and conscience or integrity that derive from their shared concern with the role that moral beliefs and values have in ethical decision making. (Given the overlap between the concepts of conscience and integrity described in Chapter 6, it is reasonable to treat them as largely interchangeable labels for a single moral domain.) The more one appreciates how close these relationships are, the more one is able to see that it is neither helpful nor accurate to speak about integrity without also speaking about ethics and moral reasoning or to speak about practical wisdom without acknowledging its dependence on foundational beliefs. If we agree that integrity fundamentally involves moral reasoning and represents the culmination of one's best efforts in moral decision making, there are important implications for medicine and medical ethics.

One of the most important of these implications is that integrity, because it integrally involves reasoning, cannot be categorized as merely a private moral experience or concern. Instead, it must be seen as something that can facilitate communication and understanding between persons and contribute to moral dialogues and debates. Though moral reasoning may arise from one person's integrity, it still has relevance for other persons. When communicated, the reasoning that pertains to one person's integrity is accessible to other persons and, thereby, open to interpersonal criticism and the possibility of revision.

[3] Reeder, "What is a religious ethic?"

Integrity entails the imperative to live life with the goal of being at unity with oneself, and in support of this goal the word *integrity* itself brings to the fore the importance of *integration* – of integrating the constellation of foundational beliefs, values, commitments, and actions that constitute our moral identities and guide our choices. Integrity refers to our need for personal wholeness and harmony, and it indicates the harm we experience when we live a double life by compartmentalizing our activities according to the multiple roles we play or social contexts we inhabit. Integrity motivates us to cultivate a single character over time and to live a life in which beliefs and actions are in harmony. Foundational beliefs are therefore an essential part of integrity, for not only do they provide the foundations of moral reasoning, but they are also inseparable from our moral identities and actions. If ethical decision making in medicine is to have genuine personal significance for physicians, those who participate in professional discussions should be ready to engage the foundational beliefs that ground a clinician's ethical judgments and determine the boundaries within which his integrity can be sustained.

Whether articulated in philosophical or religious terms, the foundational beliefs and associated values that define a professional's integrity are diverse, definitive, and decisive. Integrity should therefore be expected to play a vital role in the determination of professionals' attitudes and practices regarding significant clinical issues, such as truth telling about medical errors, respect for patient autonomy toward the end of life, and the meaning of human dignity in advanced dementia. The pre-professional worldviews that clinicians bring to their practices should be expected to exert heavy influence on their responses to such issues. Like all other persons, health care professionals need integrity and should be treated as morally autonomous persons who must decide for themselves which moral beliefs, values, and traditions are authoritative for them. Their decisions will be made within a lively network of moral interaction created by the beliefs, values, and traditions of their patients, colleagues, and society.

But in the midst of this lively network, from the perspective of each clinician there is a moral reality, individual integrity – that constellation of foundational beliefs, values, commitments, and actions that provides moral identity, defines greatest purposes, and guides choices. It is in light of this reality that the framework for practical wisdom offered here is described as *integrity-centered* and, as such, places the clinician's integrity at the moral center of the clinician's decision making. An integrity-centered ethics should not be taken to mean a self-centered ethics, but rather to imply that ethics for each individual must begin and end with each individual's deepest and most enduring beliefs and values. As an indication of how un-self-centered integrity can and (we may hope) should be, one need only look to clinicians whose integrity leads to self-sacrificial, rather than self-serving, behavior – such as those who care for patients during an epidemic at risk to their own lives or those who devote a large amount of uncompensated time to their patients or to the training and mentoring of students and young professionals. When we see examples of professional service that come at a personal cost – whether of physical or emotional health, family well-being, financial opportunity, or time – we are reminded of the remarkable commitment that integrity can motivate. The interdependence between a professional's integrity and her motivation for professional service – which is at the heart of conscientious practice – should not be underestimated.

E. Motivation and Action

It is right to assume that a characteristic feature of having a moral belief is having the inclination to act on it. It would be strange, for example, to hold the moral belief that lying is wrong and then proceed to act as though truth telling does not matter or is simply an option rather than an expectation or requirement. To believe that something is right or wrong, or good or bad, is to indicate that one is committed to living in accordance with that belief. To do otherwise would reflect flippancy, incoherence, or hypocrisy. One of the distinctive strengths of virtue ethics is that it makes the concordance between belief and action explicit in the moral life. To have a virtue, such as honesty, means that one's character includes a disposition and a desire to live out that virtue by speaking truthfully and avoiding deception. Virtues integrate thinking and feeling by combining knowledge of what is right with taking pleasure in doing it. In this way virtue ethics places motivation at the heart of the moral life and thereby bridges the potential gap between knowing and doing by insisting that it is not enough to know or believe what is right, since one must also have the intention to act according to that knowledge or belief.

When integrity is viewed three-dimensionally as involving moral reasoning, moral emotion, and moral motivation, it implicitly makes the will to act inseparable from the conclusions of reason. This relationship between will and reason parallels the relationship between motivation and deliberation found in the virtue of practical wisdom. The framework for practical wisdom in medicine offered here entails motivation toward action because practical wisdom is a virtue and because moral reasoning and integrity call for a basic harmony between what we believe and what we do. Seen this way, practical wisdom in medicine and ethics is never merely an intellectual exercise; it is ultimately action-oriented and deeply personal.

II. FOSTERING PRACTICAL WISDOM IN MEDICINE AMID MORAL PLURALISM

Practical wisdom in medicine depends on the moral beliefs and values that clinicians bring to their professional work. This dependence is most obvious when there is a need to decide which goals of medicine, goals of care, virtues, and principles should serve as the guiding objectives and moral standards of patient care and how these should be specified and prioritized in specific cases. The moral content within the framework for practical wisdom requires specification and affirmation by individuals to achieve the individual ownership that moral integrity requires. Once a person fills this or any other moral framework with particular moral content, that person must reckon with the moral diversity of the persons and communities with whom he interacts. Engaging this diversity in Western societies can test the consensus that democracies rely on to maintain shared commitments to moral expectations, policies, and laws. Though the practice of medicine enjoys a substantial degree of moral consensus concerning the pursuit of health and healing, the challenges of moral pluralism are nevertheless real for health care professionals and in some contexts can pose serious moral tensions and conflicts.

As previously mentioned, the problem of moral pluralism cannot be resolved by the supposition of a morally neutral vantage point. Nor can the problem be set aside by references to public reason, since all rationality is situated and dependent on basic beliefs that are not amenable to proof outside of the presupposed rational frameworks that support them. The suggestion of the idea of public reason is also problematic because it fails to respect the human need to live in ways that express the comprehensive belief systems (religious or philosophical) that define our lives and are consciously integrated with our choices and actions.[4] Given the dependence of practical wisdom on moral beliefs and values that are bound to be diverse in morally pluralistic societies, it is important to consider the kinds of personal, professional, and social resources that may

[4] Audi and Wolterstorff, *Religion in the public square*, 116.

be able to facilitate shared decision making, professional cooperation, and respectful social engagement and accommodation. The resources on which I focus are interpersonal communication, moral imagination, humility, professional education, and social deliberation.

A. Interpersonal Communication

Given what has been said about the implications of moral pluralism for an integrity-centered account of medicine and ethics, the proposed framework for practical wisdom poses special challenges for communication. In the routine course of shared decision making, clinicians make recommendations based on their understanding of patients' biomedical conditions and personal preferences. They should be expected to explain the rationale for such recommendations so there is mutual understanding among patients, families, and other involved professionals. These explanations are typically expressed in biomedical and technical terms, with an emphasis on risks and benefits as part of informed consent. When decision making is perceived as routine, underlying ethical assumptions are likely to be taken for granted and left unstated. But when shared decision making uncovers contrasting or conflicting perspectives about a patient's best interests, it is to be expected that ethical reasons should enter directly into conversations between physicians, patients, and families. Without the articulation of ethical reasoning, there is unlikely to be an understanding of the beliefs and values that underlie conflicting perspectives. How ethical reasons for pursuing a given course of action are given and explained then becomes significant. If these dialogues arc to be marked by mutual respect and understanding, they will require not only candor, but also moral imagination and humility, as noted later.

But there are three other reasons for the importance of moral dialogue, especially when serious disagreements arise. The first of these, as Charles Taylor explains, is the fundamentally *dialogical* character of moral life that gives interpersonal moral dialogue special relevance for moral identity.[5] On this view, as we communicate our beliefs and values to others in moral dialogues, we also increase our moral understanding of ourselves. Through dialogue, our moral identities are cultivated and sustained, and the act of articulating our beliefs and reasons strengthens our pursuit of the good that our beliefs and reasons represent. In the professional context, as clinicians articulate their reasons for pursuing a given course

[5] Taylor, *The ethics of authenticity*, 33–35.

of action – or living a certain kind of integrated life – their listeners are informed, their own reasons are opened to critical dialogue, and their own moral identities are strengthened. Seen this way, moral dialogue is a formative interpersonal engagement and a vital component of an active professional community.

A second reason for candid moral dialogue stems from the fallible nature of conscience (or integrity). If conscience involves practical moral reasoning, then it can err because of mistakes in observation, interpretation of facts, or assessment of the moral values pertinent to those facts. Conscience can also be misled by self-deception and rationalization. Mistakes in moral reasoning, weaknesses in moral character, and self-deception explain why conscience should never be treated as if it were beyond dialogue and questioning, even if in the end it is respected as being finally authoritative for each individual.

A third reason arises from the substantial connection between integrity or conscience and practical moral reasoning. Because the function of integrity entails reasoning, it is not relevant merely to the individual whose integrity is at issue. Moral reasoning that arises from deliberations about integrity serves as a communicative bridge from one person to another. Thus, the normative reach of integrity is not limited to the private realm of one individual, but carries meaning – when articulated by reasoning – for others in the professional or civic communities in which that individual works and lives. Dialogues regarding matters of integrity benefit these communities and also lessen the potential for inordinate individualism by placing the subjective authority of integrity in a context of mutual accountability.

This accountability can create an equilibrium in which a group helps form the integrity of its individual members, while individuals both sustain and challenge the moral practices and standards of the group. Within professional communities, the habit of moral dialogue between colleagues fosters a culture of moral calibration through which individual clinicians help, and are helped by, the ethos of their peers as together they engage in testing, reinforcing, and refining each other's moral assumptions, conclusions, priorities, and practices. By engaging in such dialogue and calibration, physicians manifest a shared moral obligation that can ground the kind of commitment to professional self-regulation that William May describes as part of a covenantal ethics for medicine.[6]

[6] William F. May, *The physician's covenant: images of the healer in medical ethics,* 2d ed. (Louisville: Westminster John Knox Press, 2000), 115, 140–48.

A relatively recent example of such self-regulation throughout the medical profession has been the widespread implementation of conflict-of-interest policies in academic medical centers.[7] The deliberations that have led to changes of policy and practice have been stimulated by forces inside and outside the medical profession, but they have included contributions from physician-leaders who speak of the importance of protecting professional integrity against threats from financial conflicts of interest that risk compromising patient care.[8]

B. Moral Imagination

In the midst of shared decision making that involves tensions or conflicts, especially when decisions are deeply personal and involve beliefs and values that reflect our moral identities, it is essential to have *moral imagination.* This is the willingness to intuit the inner lives of those around us, to "develop an ability to be aware of others as persons, as important to themselves as we are to ourselves, and to have a lively and sympathetic representation in imagination of their interests and of the effects of our actions on their lives."[9] The morally imaginative clinician is one who tries to understand the patient's uniqueness as clearly as possible, endeavoring to perceive what the patient values most deeply. Moral imagination can be seen as the perceptiveness that is necessary for responding altruistically to the needs of a patient. When a physician understands a patient's needs in the context of the patient's deeper beliefs and values, she will be all the more capable of treating the patient with sensitivity to the ways in which the clinical encounter, its deliberations, and its decisions may affect the patient as the person he is – even if there are disagreements between them that cannot be resolved. Moral imagination is closely related to what has been called the *moral point of view* – a moral perspective that allows one to reach an ethical conclusion that is sufficiently considered and rigorous. Its characteristics indicate what "doing ethics" essentially entails and can be listed as follows:

7 Rothman and Chimonas, "New developments in managing physician–industry relationships."

8 T. A. Brennan et al., "Health industry practices that create conflicts of interest: a policy proposal for academic medical centers," *JAMA* 295 (2006): 429–33.

9 Frankena, *Ethics,* 69.

1. concern for how one's own actions affect the lives of other persons;[10]
2. at a basic level, equal treatment for everyone[11] in the sense of equal worth and respect for human dignity;[12]
3. impartiality in the pursuit of fairness and a refusal to make exceptions for one's own case;[13]
4. reliance on reasoning and the willingness to universalize one's moral judgments so that conclusions apply to all persons in the same situation;[14] and
5. the ability to place oneself in the role of other persons (i.e., Kohlberg's reversibility, which can be seen as a kind of moral musical chairs).[15]

The fifth characteristic suggests a link between ethics and empathy. In the clinical context, empathy focuses on the emotional dynamic between a patient and a clinician.[16] But it also entails "perspective-taking,"[17] which is "a cognitive capacity to take the perspective of the other person while keeping self and other differentiated."[18] By attending to the cognitive work of perspective-taking, empathy can be seen as directly relevant to the moral imagination a clinician needs when making decisions with patients, families, and other clinicians. These five characteristics, if adopted in the course of shared decision making about morally contested issues, can be expected to go a long way in cushioning the impact of disagreements and identifying paths toward their reconciliation.

C. Humility

Moral deliberation in medicine also calls for humility. In the context of an integrity-centered framework for practical wisdom that takes moral pluralism into account, humility assumes special moral significance. In

[10] Ibid., 113.
[11] Nagel, "Moral conflict and political legitimacy."
[12] Nussbaum, *Liberty of conscience*, 56.
[13] Ibid.; Nagel, "Moral conflict and political legitimacy."
[14] Callahan, *In good conscience*, 28; Frankena, *Ethics*, 113.
[15] Langston, *Conscience and other virtues*, 163.
[16] Jodi Halpern, "Clinical empathy in medical care," in *Empathy: from bench to bedside*, ed. Jean Decety (Cambridge, MA: MIT Press, 2012), 229–44.
[17] Johanna Shapiro, "The paradox of teaching empathy in medical education," in *Empathy*, ed. Decety, 283.
[18] Philip L. Jackson, Andrew N. Meltzoff, and Jean Decety, "How do we perceive the pain of others? A window into the neural processes involved in empathy," *NeuroImage* 24 (2005): 771–79.

Chapter 3 it was observed that practical wisdom involves a humble openness to the world as it is, in contrast to cunning or cleverness, by which one attempts to impose self-serving intentions onto the world through deception or manipulation. In Chapter 5 it was observed that the existence of fallibility in the function of conscience creates a pressing need for a humility that encourages moral imagination and self-scrutiny. Even when an individual is compelled by conscience to stand firm in the strength of her moral convictions, humility encourages confidence without arrogance, a distinction that was perhaps one of the most impressive character traits of Abraham Lincoln.[19] Humility can also foster a spirit of tolerance in a pluralistic democracy by countering the tendency of human pride to hide the finite character of human endeavors and their susceptibility to error.[20]

D. Professional Education

Practical wisdom and other virtues present a major challenge for education. As acquired traits, virtues are learned through experience and practice, not by attending lectures or taking online tutorials. Acquiring virtues is a process of habituation nourished by practice and reflection within a virtue-supporting community that encourages its members to pursue and find satisfaction in what is agreed to be good. Development in virtue involves a growing harmony between a person's moral attitudes, feelings, and judgments, and the *desire* to grow in virtue is essential for progress. The formative role of a community that cultivates the virtues draws attention to the problem of the "hidden curriculum"[21] – that is, those aspects of the learning environment that instill negative values instead of virtues. The hidden curriculum makes clear that the learning environment is vulnerable to virtue-suppressing influences. Deliberate efforts are needed to make this environment as virtue-enhancing as possible, through role modeling, shared expectations, and the implementation of organizational structures and institutional policies that reinforce the formal curriculum of ethics rather than undermine it. Such efforts ought to include leaders who are respected not only for their research,

[19] William Lee Miller, *Lincoln's virtues: an ethical biography* (New York: Knopf, 2002), 293.

[20] Niebuhr, *The children of light and the children of darkness*, 134–35.

[21] Hafferty and Franks, "The hidden curriculum, ethics teaching, and the structure of medical education."

clinical skills, and teaching skills, but also for their moral values and concern for the moral life of their professional communities.

The framework for practical wisdom offered in this book recognizes that practical wisdom in medicine depends on the moral beliefs and values to which clinicians are committed and by which they decide what goals, virtues, and principles they will follow. As such, training in practical wisdom cannot be detached from training in ethics or from an awareness of the relationship between moral reasoning and moral integrity. Professionals need to come to terms with the beliefs, values, and goals that form the normative standards that will guide their practice as they respond to the needs of patients and the expectations of professional organizations, health care institutions, and society.

Identifying the normative standards that should guide one's practice of medicine can be seen as part of a trainee's responsibility to engage in the process of moral formation by which integrity is developed. This process includes a willingness to refine, reform, and prioritize one's moral beliefs and values in light of moral resources that include a trainee's prior moral commitments, recognized standards of ethics and professionalism, lessons of experience, and the testing and reinforcement that come from dialogue within a moral community. And the process of moral formation will reflect a continuous integration of moral reasons, moral emotions, and moral action – all motivated by a desire to live what is believed to be a good life and to make decisions on the basis of what that goodness entails. This formation is aided by humility – that self-scrutinizing and teachable attitude that motivates one to emulate role models, learn from mistakes, acknowledge prejudices, and modify judgments in light of new information or better insights.

E. Social Deliberation and Legal Limits

An accurate perception of medicine's moral landscape reveals three directions of moral responsibility that represent the patient's good, the professional's integrity, and society's needs. These responsibilities can be seen as a triangle held intact by mutually reinforcing commitments and expectations. From the perspective of the health professional, the stability of the triangle necessarily depends on the professional's moral integrity, for a professional's integrity not only preserves his moral identity, but also sustains his commitments to patients and to society. This shows why it is so edifying for professionals when the triangle of responsibility is held together by mutually reinforcing expectations of patients, professionals, and society and why, in contrast, it is so problematic when the triangle is destabilized by conflicts among the expectations of patients, professionals, and society.

Seen through the lens of the "social contract," society grants the medical profession special privileges and, in return, expects certain benefits. An interpretation of the contract that favors greater degrees of control over physicians adopts a social constructivist view of the medical profession, claiming its members are like civil servants, obligated to provide all legally available medical services. An interpretation that favors greater degrees of physician autonomy views medical professionals as guardians of a practice who are entitled to establish the boundaries of professional obligation based on their assessments of health and disease and the internal goods that medicine is supposed to advance. Interpretations that are more autonomy-respecting resonate with an integrity-centered practice of medicine, as they view physicians as morally autonomous persons whose individual convictions – derived from professional, philosophical, and religious beliefs – create interpretive frameworks by which medicine's purposes are understood and its boundaries defined and preserved.

Within the social contract, physicians voluntarily assume commitments that create special responsibilities, which include altruistic service, respect for patient autonomy, commitment to high ethical standards, promotion of the public good, and acceptance of reimbursement mechanisms and cost-controlling policies. Sometimes society justifiably exercises its prerogatives within the social contract in response to physician behaviors that disregard generally accepted features of a health professional's fiduciary responsibilities. This can be seen, for example, in federal and state regulatory responses to conflicts of interest arising from financial relationships between physicians and health care companies. Some commentators see these relationships as creating ethical risks;[22] others would add that financial relationships may also reflect unethical motives.[23] Whether due to ethically dangerous circumstances or ethically suspect motivations, conflicts of interest among physicians illustrate the limitations of relying on individual physician virtue or conscience as the sole safeguard of patient welfare. The emergence of conflict-of-interest policies and regulations indicates that at times society finds it necessary to direct physicians, by persuasion or requirement, away from practices that may or do compromise the fulfillment of physicians' fiduciary obligations.

[22] Institute of Medicine, *Conflict of interest in medical research, education, and practice*, 46–49.
[23] Brennan et al., "Health industry practices that create conflicts of interest."

But in other contexts – such as abortion, contraception, or physician-assisted suicide – some clinicians may believe that the expectations of society impose inappropriate demands that contradict moral commitments they perceive to be of primary importance. In such cases, there is the prospect of deep tension between society's prerogative to impose its will on medicine and the medical professional's prerogative to practice medicine with integrity. Within a morally pluralistic society, such tension will be less likely to emerge if there is widespread agreement about which clinical practices should be considered controversial and therefore deserving of policy and legal mechanisms to accommodate freedom of practice.

The most formal manifestations of such accommodations are conscience clauses in federal and state laws. These can provide important legal protections for health care professionals whose foundational beliefs prevent them from providing, participating in, or referring patients for certain morally contested but legally available medical services. They also reflect society's acknowledgment of the deeply controversial nature of some medical services and its commitment to honor liberty of conscience among all citizens, including health care professionals. However, the sticking point for the implementation of conscience clauses will always be the challenge of determining whether a given practice should be considered controversial in the first place. And that challenge will usually center on deciding what threats to the liberty of one person (i.e., a patient) might justify placing legal constraints on the liberty and conscience of another (i.e., a physician). There will always be a need for professional, social, and political deliberation to determine where the boundaries of individual professional freedom of conscience should be drawn. Depending on prevailing laws, in some circumstances clinicians who act on the courage of their convictions to preserve their moral integrity may have to be willing to suffer penalties for doing so.

If one adopts a *physician-respecting standard* to assess conflicts that arise from conscientious refusals by physicians, one can acknowledge the physician's prima facie obligation to respect and promote a patient's treatment preferences without minimizing the need to respect and protect the professional's conscience in matters that are controversial. This standard reflects the belief that both patients and physicians have moral autonomy that merits respect, implying that neither the patient nor the physician should be allowed to override the conscience of the other. This mutual respect for autonomy and conscience may be criticized on the grounds that the patient–physician relationship is asymmetrical with respect to purpose, power, and knowledge. These are significant issues to consider. Even so, concerns about asymmetry can be addressed by acknowledging the need for serious unilateral obligations on physicians to care for and respect patients, while also recognizing that respect for patient autonomy should never be treated as if it were a justification for limitless deference to patient preferences.

Moral disputes involving medical professionals frequently emphasize the *negative* work of conscience and are cast in terms of *conscientious objection.* But the reasoning, feelings, and motivation that constitute conscience not only repel one away from morally objectionable actions, but also draw one toward morally desirable goals. Conscience therefore also does *positive* work, as signified by the notion of *conscientious practice* that captures the interdependence between a professional's conscience and her motivation for service as a health care practitioner. This motivation lies at the heart of an integrity-centered practice of medicine, and it warrants enduring respect and cultivation if medical professionals are to be encouraged to integrate medicine and ethics in the care of their patients.

III. IMPLICATIONS OF PRACTICAL WISDOM FOR CLINICAL PRACTICE: FOUR ILLUSTRATIONS

The framework for practical wisdom in medicine this book offers should make it clear that the way physicians respond to ethical challenges in medicine depends on what they believe and value. Moral reasoning and moral action rely on choices about goals, perception of moral values and moral responsibilities, and prioritization of principles and virtues. And a physician's response to an ethical challenge will depend on his integrity, that is, on his beliefs and values as they pertain to goals, responsibilities, and priorities, and the degree to which his actions are consistent with those beliefs and values.

In passing, it is useful to make a point about the relationship between consistency and integrity. Common use of the term *integrity* implies that it is always a good thing. We automatically assume that someone who acts with integrity is to be commended. This routinely positive attitude carries a further assumption that the beliefs and values guiding such action are also morally praiseworthy. It is because beliefs, values, and actions are all laudable in a given case that consistency between them is seen as representing the positive attribute we call integrity. But it is important to note, of course, that mere consistency between beliefs, values, and actions does not guarantee moral praiseworthiness, for if any of the beliefs and values in question were thought to be morally objectionable, then the opposite would likely be true. One can look at historical examples of injustice to see that evil deeds have at times been perpetrated under the influence of beliefs, values, and actions that were consistent, but terribly bad. Mention of integrity should always invite questions about moral content and prompt discussion and assessment of the beliefs, values, and actions involved – which will always bring one back to moral reasoning.

To illustrate how integrity depends on specific beliefs and values, perceptions about goals, responsibilities, and the prioritization of principles and virtues, it is helpful to consider examples. To this end, I offer brief descriptions of four clinical situations that indicate how clinical circumstances challenge health professionals to decide what they believe and value and that reveal how those beliefs and values determine the moral substance of integrity and its impact on decision making.

Physician-assisted suicide is a controversial practice that continues to raise ethical and policy concerns even though it has been legalized in some European countries and a few states in America.[24] This practice – in which a physician intentionally prescribes a lethal dose of medication that a patient can take in order to commit suicide – raises fundamental questions about the goals of medicine, the boundaries of palliative care, the meaning and expression of compassion, the nature of a physician's obligation to respond to suffering, the moral significance of causes and intentions when the outcome of death is assumed to be inevitable, the moral status of suicide, the scope of a patient's freedom and autonomy, and the prerogative of a physician's conscientious practice. Though some of these questions are specific to assisted suicide, others arise commonly in the context of end-of-life care, especially after physicians, patients, and families have decided that the patient's most important goal of care is being comfortable, not living longer. Physicians who are involved in decision making with patients and families toward the end of life cannot avoid the need to rely on assumptions, based on their beliefs and values, regarding a range of serious issues: the goals of care that are deemed appropriate at a given point of time; the responsibilities they have to the patient, the family, themselves, and society; the principles (such as respect for patient autonomy, beneficence, and nonmaleficence) and virtues (such as compassion and courage) that are deemed most important;

[24] Lois Snyder and Daniel P. Sulmasy, "Physician-assisted suicide (American College of Physicians position paper)," *Annals of Internal Medicine* 135 (2001): 209–16.

how those principles and virtues will be understood and prioritized; and whether certain actions should be considered intrinsically wrong (such as intentionally causing or hastening death). The context of end-of-life care teems with moral questions that will be answered, whether the answers are explicitly articulated or implicitly enacted. How physicians respond to the needs and requests of patients and families will depend on the beliefs and values they bring to this context.

Another clinical situation that provokes some of the questions just mentioned is *Alzheimer dementia*. As this condition worsens, persons experience a range of progressively debilitating symptoms, both physical and cognitive.[25] When persons with dementia are no longer able to make their own medical decisions, their surrogate decision makers have to assume responsibility for deciding what treatments are appropriate as the condition worsens and as complications arise.[26] Making these decisions depends on surrogates' perceptions of what their loved ones would have wanted, assessments of the relative benefits of survival and quality of life, assumptions about what defines personhood and dignity for human beings, beliefs about what makes a life worth living, and considerations related to the emotional, time, and economic burdens of caregiving. Physicians who work with surrogate decision makers in deciding what life-sustaining treatments should be provided will bring to these decisions their own constellations of assumptions, assessments, and beliefs regarding the issues just mentioned, and they will presumably have ideas (spoken or not) about the extent to which society should bear the financial costs of supporting the use of life-sustaining procedures for persons in moderate or advanced stages of dementia. As physicians and surrogate decision makers face decisions about life-sustaining treatments – for example, resuscitation procedures in the case of cardiac arrest, admissions to acute care hospitals to treat intermittent complications, or antibiotics to treat urinary tract infections or pneumonias – the assumptions and judgments of surrogates, physicians, and other health professionals will combine to guide the decisions that are made.

A very different kind of clinical situation arises when there is a need for the *disclosure of medical errors*. Medical errors are an unfortunate reality for patients and clinicians alike, and efforts to decrease errors represent

[25] A. C. Hurley and L. Volicer, "Alzheimer disease: 'It's okay, Mama, if you want to go, it's okay,'" *JAMA* 288 (2002): 2324–31.

[26] Lauris C. Kaldjian et al., "Dementia, goals of care, and personhood: a study of surrogate decision makers' beliefs and values," *American Journal of Hospice and Palliative Medicine* 27 (2010): 387–97.

a high priority in current health care practices.[27] After an error occurs, physicians should take steps to disclose the error and should do so to patients and their families as part of patient care,[28] to hospitals for the sake of improving patient safety,[29] and to colleagues in order to enhance professional learning.[30] But the process of deciding whether, how, and when to disclose errors in these three "directions" can be extremely demanding, given how devastating it can be for physicians to be involved in an error, especially when it results in grave harm to a patient. There are numerous factors that facilitate physicians' willingness to communicate about errors, but there are also many factors that can impede that willingness.[31] Facilitating factors include virtues and motivations such as honesty, respectfulness, accountability, courage, altruism, empathy, humility, acceptance of fallibility, and the desire for forgiveness and reconciliation. Impeding factors include pride, arrogance, self-interest, and a host of fears related to loss of trust, loss of reputation, and possible professional, financial, and legal repercussions. Given how many reasons there can be to remain silent after an error has been made, it is essential for a physician to have compelling reasons to do the hard but necessary work of disclosure, and this involves having a clear view of the goals of disclosure, endorsing the moral responsibilities at stake (to patients, to fellow professionals, and to society), and being committed to the principles and virtues that support disclosure. If a physician's integrity includes a commitment to these goals, responsibilities, principles, and virtues, she will take the steps necessary to see to it that an error is disclosed. In doing so, she will display what conscientious practice can mean when it motivates action under painfully uncomfortable circumstances.

Yet another clinical challenge arises when physicians and other health care professionals are called upon to *care for infectious patients during times of epidemic.* This situation can create an enormous strain on clinicians, hospitals, and communities that may result in tensions between the interests of professionals, the patients they serve, the institutions in which they

[27] L. T. Kohn, J. M. Corrigan, and M. S. Donaldson, *To err is human: building a safer health system* (Washington, DC: National Academy Press, 2000).

[28] Lauris C. Kaldjian et al., "Disclosing medical errors to patients: attitudes and practices of physicians and trainees," *Journal of General Internal Medicine* 22 (2007): 988–96.

[29] Lauris C. Kaldjian et al., "Reporting medical errors to improve patient safety: a survey of physicians in teaching hospitals," *Archives of Internal Medicine* 168 (2008): 40–46.

[30] Lauris C. Kaldjian et al., "Do faculty and resident physicians discuss their medical errors?" *Journal of Medical Ethics* 34 (2008): 717–22.

[31] Kaldjian et al., "An empirically derived taxonomy of factors affecting physicians' willingness to disclose medical errors."

work and the public's health. Though some would say there is professional and social consensus about a health professional's duty to serve in time of epidemic,[32] others would suggest that experience reveals a lack of consensus among professionals about the extent to which altruism should be expected of them, as witnessed by disagreements about how much professionals should be willing to sacrifice of their and their families' interests in order to protect the public's health.[33] When service comes at a personal risk and family cost, it will inevitably be guided by the goals of medicine that clinicians perceive to be most compelling, the moral responsibilities believed to have highest priority (to patients, to the public, to themselves, or to their families), and the principles (such as beneficence and utility) and virtues (such as courage, altruism, and fidelity to family) believed to be most relevant amid a web of competing obligations. As in the case of error disclosure, duty to serve during an epidemic demands that health care professionals rely on moral beliefs and values that reflect some of the highest moral standards in medicine. Those who hold such beliefs and values, and try to make their actions consistent with them, will be acting with integrity and illustrating what conscientious practice can look like in one of its most self-giving forms.

IV. CONCLUDING REMARKS

The beliefs and values physicians bring to their clinical encounters will inevitably determine the way they think, speak, and act. And this will bear heavily on the outcomes of decisions that physicians make with patients and families. There is no way around this reality. Outcomes of decision making depend on the particularities physicians bring to the practice of medicine.

The framework for practical wisdom in medicine offered in this chapter can be seen as a way of taking this reality seriously by bringing into the open the beliefs, values, and reasoning that influence, one way or another, the process of clinical decision making. This framework asks us to be deliberate about the goals that guide clinical care. It asks us to perceive patients and their circumstances accurately by inquiring about their goals and their

[32] J. G. Bartlett, "Planning for avian influenza," *Annals of Internal Medicine* 145 (2006): 141–44.

[33] P. A. Singer et al., "Ethics and SARS: lessons from Toronto," *British Medical Journal* 327 (2003): 1342–44.

assessments of the probabilities and burdens associated with their care. It directs our attention not only to patients, but also to our own integrity and the needs of society. It appreciates the complementary roles of principles and virtues. It recognizes that ethical reasoning should be part of conscience, not separate from it, and that integrity – if it is to fulfill its deeper meaning – requires moral integration that leads to wholeness in our lives. And it acknowledges that good reasoning and right thinking will be powerless without the motivation to act on what is believed to be good and right.

When in the course of her work a physician has occasion to refer to her integrity or conscience as the basis for a decision, that reference sends a signal to her listeners that she has foundational beliefs and values at stake that need to be taken very seriously. In the health professions and in society, we do well to interpret claims of integrity or conscience as indicators of a degree of moral seriousness that reaches to the level of moral identity. Unpacking these foundational beliefs and values may sometimes be necessary so that patients, families, colleagues, and perhaps society can understand the moral reasoning that is an essential part of what is being put forward when claims of integrity or conscience are made. These claims are best seen as invitations to engage in dialogue about the beliefs, values, and ethical reasoning that guide a clinician's decision making. Through dialogue we may hope that all people involved will better understand the moral reasons being communicated in the name of integrity or conscience and why those reasons carry such potent meaning for the one who expresses them.

To navigate through the ordinary and extraordinary ethical challenges of medical practice, clinicians need practical wisdom to discern, integrate, and decide between the contrasting moral goods and competing claims that can arise in clinical decision making. We can encourage growth toward such wisdom in the medical community by teaching, modeling, and practicing medicine in ways that integrate goals of care, clear perception, accurate information, core principles and virtues, moral reasoning, integrity, motivation, and action. We can also try to foster in each other the habits of respectful communication, moral imagination, and humility – habits that enhance decisions shared by clinicians, patients, and families and that facilitate constructive dialogue when moral disagreements arise.

I do not deny that the achievement of practical wisdom in medicine is a great aspiration. But over the years I have been privileged to know physicians who have displayed such wisdom. This observation is not only inspiring but also reassuring, for it confirms that wisdom in medicine is a very real possibility. Yet the observation also stands as a challenge, for such exemplars remind me that I, too, can continue to endeavor toward the same. Whether I will make that endeavor my own depends not only on who I am, but on who I would like to be.

Bibliography

AAP, Committee on Bioethics. "Policy statement: physician refusal to provide information or treatment on the basis of claims of conscience." *Pediatrics* 124 (2009): 1689–93.

ABIM Foundation (American Board of Internal Medicine). "Medical professionalism in the new millennium: a physician charter." *Annals of Internal Medicine* 136 (2002): 243–46.

ACOG, Committee on Ethics. "End-of-life decision making (committee report no. 403)." *Obstetrics and Gynecology* 111 (2008): 1021–27.

"End-of-life decision making: understanding goals of care." *International Journal of Gynecology & Obstetrics* 50 (1995): 208–14.

"The limits of conscientious refusal in reproductive medicine (committee opinion no. 385)." *Obstetrics and Gynecology* 110 (2007): 1203–1208.

"Medical futility (committee opinion no. 362)." *Obstetrics and Gynecology* 109 (2007): 791–94.

ACP. *American College of Physicians ethics manual*, 6th ed. Philadelphia: American College of Physicians, 2012.

"How can our nation conserve and distribute health care resources effectively and efficiently?" Philadelphia: American College of Physicians, 2011.

Althaus, Paul. *The ethics of Martin Luther*. Philadelphia: Fortress Press, 1972.

AMA, Code of Medical Ethics. "Opinion 2.035: futile care." American Medical Association, 1994. www.ama-assn.org/ama/pub/physician-resources/medical-ethics/code-medical-ethics/opinion2035.page.

"Opinion 2.037: medical futility in end-of-life care." American Medical Association, 1997. www.ama-assn.org/ama/pub/physician-resources/medical-ethics/code-medical-ethics/opinion2037.page.

"Opinion 9.067: physician obligation in disaster preparedness and response." American Medical Association, 2004. www.ama-assn.org/ama/pub/physician-resources/medical-ethics/code-medical-ethics/opinion9067.page.

"Opinion 10.05: potential patients." American Medical Association, 2008. www.ama-assn.org/ama/pub/physician-resources/medical-ethics/code-medical-ethics/opinion1005.page.

AMA, Council on Judicial Affairs. "Physician objection to treatment and individual patient discrimination (CEJA report no. 6-a-07)." American Medical Association, 2007.

ANA. "American Nurses Association Code of Ethics." American Nurses Association, 2001.

Annas, Julia. *The morality of happiness.* Oxford: Oxford University Press, 1993.

Aquinas, Thomas. *Summa theologica: a concise translation.* Translated by Timothy McDermott. Westminster, MD: Christian Classics, 1989.

Aristotle. *Nicomachean ethics.* Translated by Martin Ostwald. Indianapolis: Bobbs-Merrill Educational Publishing, 1962.

Association of American Medical Colleges. *In the interest of patients: recommendations for physician financial relationships and clinical decision making.* Washington, DC, 2010.

Audi, Robert, and Nicholas Wolterstorff. *Religion in the public square.* Lanham, MD: Rowman & Littlefield, 1997.

Bainton, Roland H. *Here I stand: a life of Martin Luther.* New York: Mentor Books, 1950.

Barth, Karl. *Church dogmatics.* Vol. III.4. Edinburgh: T. & T. Clark, 1961.

Bartlett, J. G. "Planning for avian influenza." *Annals of Internal Medicine* 145 (2006): 141–44.

Beauchamp, Tom L. "What's so special about the virtues?" In *Virtue and medicine.* Edited by Earl E. Shelp. 307–27. Dordrecht: Reidel, 1985.

Beauchamp, Tom L., and James F. Childress. *Principles of biomedical ethics.* 6th ed. New York: Oxford University Press, 2009.

Benjamin, Martin. *Splitting the difference: compromise and integrity in ethics and politics.* Lawrence: University Press of Kansas, 1990.

Bible. New International Version. Grand Rapids, MI: Zondervan, 1996.

Bleich, J. David. "The physician as a conscientious objector." *Fordham Urban Law Journal* 30 (2002): 245–65.

Blustein, Jeffrey. "Doing what the patient orders: maintaining integrity in the doctor–patient relationship." *Bioethics* 7, no. 4 (1993): 289–314.

Bonhoeffer, Dietrich. *Ethics.* New York: Macmillan, 1955.

Bostock, David. *Aristotle's ethics.* Oxford: Oxford University Press, 2000.

Brennan, Michael D. "Professionalism and academic medicine: the Mayo Clinic program in professionalism." *Irish Journal of Medical Science* 177 (2008): 23–27.

Brennan, T. A., D. J. Rothman, L. Blank, D. Blumenthal, S. C. Chimonas, J. J. Cohen, J. Goldman, et al. "Health industry practices that create conflicts of interest: a policy proposal for academic medical centers." *JAMA* 295 (2006): 429–33.

Broad, C. D. "Conscience and conscientious action." In *Conscience.* Edited by John Donnelly and Leonard Lyons. 5–23. Staten Island, NY: Alba House, 1973.

Brock, Dan W. "Conscientious refusal by physicians and pharmacists: who is obligated to do what, and why?" *Theoretical Medicine and Bioethics* 29 (2008): 187–200.

"Facts and values in the physician–patient relationship." In *Ethics, trust, and the professions: philosophical and cultural aspects.* Edited by E. D. Pellegrino, R. M. Veatch, and J. P. Langan. 113–30. Washington, DC: Georgetown University Press, 1991.

Butler, Joseph. *Five sermons.* Indianapolis: Hackett, 1983.

Cahill, Lisa Sowle. "Theology and bioethics: should religious traditions have a public voice?" *Journal of Medicine and Philosophy* 17 (1992): 263–72.

Callahan, Sidney. *In good conscience: reason and emotion in moral decision making.* New York: HarperCollins, 1991.

Calvin, John. *Institutes of the Christian religion.* Edited by John T. McNeill. Philadelphia: Westminster Press, 1960.

Campbell, Courtney S. "Bearing witness: religious resistance and meaning." In *Notes from a narrow ridge: religion and bioethics.* Edited by Dena S. Davis and Laurie Zoloth. 21–48. Hagerstown, MD: University Publishing Group, 1999.

"Religion and Moral Meaning in Bioethics." *Hastings Center Report* 20, no. 4 (1990): S4–S10.

Campbell, Courtney S., Jan Hare, and Pam Matthews. "Conflicts of conscience: hospice and assisted suicide." *Hastings Center Report* 25, no. 3 (1995): 36–43.

Cantor, J. D. "Conscientious objection gone awry: restoring selfless professionalism in medicine." *New England Journal of Medicine* 360 (2009): 1484–85.

Cantor, Julie, and Ken Baum. "The limits of conscientious objection: may pharmacists refuse to fill prescriptions for emergency contraception?" *New England Journal of Medicine* 351 (2004): 2008–12.

Cassel, Christine K., and Sachin H. Jain. "Assessing individual physician performance: does measurement suppress motivation?" *JAMA* 307, no. 24 (2012): 2595–96.

Charo, R. A. "The celestial fire of conscience: refusing to deliver medical care." *New England Journal of Medicine* 352 (2005): 2471–73.

Chervenak, Frank A., and Laurence B. McCullough. "An ethically justified practical approach to offering, recommending, performing, and referring for induced abortion and feticide." *American Journal of Obstetrics and Gynecology* 201 (2009): 560.e1–6.

Childress, James F. "Appeals to conscience." *Ethics* 89 (1979): 315–35.

"Conscience and conscientious actions in the context of MCOs." *Kennedy Institute of Ethics Journal* 7 (1997): 403–11.

Chimonas, S. C., T. A. Brennan, and D. J. Rothman. "Physicians and drug representatives: exploring the dynamics of the relationship." *Journal of General Internal Medicine* 22 (2007): 184–90.

Cohen, Henry. "The evolution of the concept of disease." In *Concepts of health and disease: interdisciplinary perspectives.* Edited by Arthur L. Caplan, H. Tristram Engelhardt, and James J. McCartney. 209–19. London: Addison-Wesley, 1981.

Cohen, Jordan J. "Linking professionalism to humanism: what it means, why it matters." *Academic Medicine* 82 (2007): 1029–32.

Combs, Michael P., Ryan M. Antiel, Jon C. Tilburt, Paul S. Mueller, and Farr A. Curlin. "Conscientious refusals to refer: findings from a national physician survey." *Journal of Medical Ethics* 37 (2011): 397–401.

"Commentary and resolution on physician assisted suicide." National Hospice & Palliative Care Organization, 2005.

Coulehan, Jack. "Today's professionalism: engaging the mind but not the heart." *Academic Medicine* 80 (2005): 892–98.

Crawshaw, Ralph, David E. Rogers, Edmund D. Pellegrino, Roger J. Bulger, George D. Lundberg, Lonnie R. Bristow, Christine K. Cassel, and Jeremiah A. Barondess. "Patient–physician covenant." *JAMA* 273 (1995): 1553.

Cruess, Richard L., and Sylvia R. Cruess. "Expectations and obligations: professionalism and medicine's social contract with society." *Perspectives in Biology and Medicine* 51, no. 4 (2008): 579–98.

Curlin, Farr A., John D. Lantos, Chad J. Roach, Sarah A. Sellergren, and Marshall H. Chin. "Religious Characteristics of U.S. Physicians: A National Survey." *Journal of General Internal Medicine* 20 (2005): 629–34.

Curlin, Farr A., Ryan E. Lawrence, Marshall H. Chin, and John D. Lantos. "Religion, conscience, and controversial clinical practices." *New England Journal of Medicine* 356 (2007): 593–600.

Curran, Charles E. "Conscience in the light of the Catholic moral tradition." In *Conscience.* Edited by Charles E. Curran. 3–24. Mahwah, NJ: Paulist Press, 2004.

D'Arcy, Eric. "Conscience." *Journal of Medical Ethics* 3 (1977): 98–99.

Conscience and its right to freedom. New York: Sheed and Ward, 1961.

Davies, Brian. *The thought of Thomas Aquinas.* Oxford: Clarendon Press, 1993.

Davis, John K. "Conscientious refusal and a doctor's right to quit." *Journal of Medicine and Philosophy* 29 (2004): 75–91.

Dickens, B. M., and R. J. Cook. "The scope and limits of conscientious objection." *International Journal of Gynecology & Obstetrics* 71 (2000): 71–77.

Diekema, Douglas S., and American Academy of Pediatrics Committee on Bioethics. "Responding to parental refusals of immunization of children." *Pediatrics* 115 (2005): 1428–31.

Dinneen, John A. "Freedom of conscience in philosophical perspective." In *Conscience: its freedom and limitations.* Edited by William C. Bier. 101–106. New York: Fordham University Press, 1971.

Dolan, Joseph V. "Conscience in the Catholic theological tradition." In *Conscience: its freedom and limitations.* Edited by William C. Bier. 9–19. New York: Fordham University Press, 1971.

Dooley, Dolores. "Conscientious refusal to assist with abortion." *British Medical Journal* 309 (1994): 622–23.

Dreisbach, Daniel L., and Mark David Hall, eds. *The sacred rights of conscience: selected readings on religious liberty and church–state relations in the American founding.* Indianapolis: Liberty Fund, 2009.

Duncan-Jones, Austin. "The notion of conscience." In *Conscience.* Edited by John Donnelly and Leonard Lyons. 115–27. Staten Island, NY: Alba House, 1973.

Elshtain, Jean Bethke. "Why Science Cannot Stand Alone." *Theoretical Medicine and Bioethics* 29 (2008): 161–69.

Elstein, Arthur S. "Human factors in clinical judgment: discussion of Scriven's 'Clinical Judgment.'" In *Clinical judgment: a critical appraisal.* Edited by H. Tristram Engelhardt, Stuart F. Spicker, and Bernard Towers. 17–28. Dordrecht: Reidel, 1979.

Engel, George L. "The need for a new medical model: a challenge for biomedicine." In *Concepts of health and disease: interdisciplinary perspectives.* Edited by Arthur L. Caplan, H. Tristram Engelhardt, and James J. McCartney. 589–607. London: Addison-Wesley, 1981.

Engelhardt, H. Tristram. "The concepts of health and disease." In *Concepts of health and disease: interdisciplinary perspectives.* Edited by Arthur L. Caplan, H. Tristram Engelhardt, and James J. McCartney. 31–45. London: Addison-Wesley, 1981.

The foundations of Christian bioethics. Lisse: Swets & Zeitlinger, 2000.

Faunce, T., S. Bolsin, and W. P. Chan. "Supporting whistleblowers in academic medicine: training and respecting the courage of professional conscience." *Journal of Medical Ethics* 30 (2004): 40–43.

Flanagan-Klygis, Erin A., Lisa Sharp, and Joel E. Frader. "Dismissing the family who refuses vaccines: a study of pediatrician attitudes." *Archives of Pediatrics and Adolescent Medicine* 159 (2005): 929–34.

Foot, Philippa. "Virtues and vices." In *Virtue ethics.* Edited by Stephen Darwall. 105–20. Oxford: Blackwell, 2003.

Frankena, William. *Ethics.* Englewood Cliffs, NJ: Prentice Hall, 1973.

Freidson, Eliot. *Profession of medicine: a study of the sociology of applied knowledge.* Chicago: University of Chicago Press, 1970.

Fuss, Peter. "Conscience." In *Conscience.* Edited by John Donnelly and Leonard Lyons. 35–50. Staten Island, NY: Alba House, 1973.

Galston, William. *Liberal purposes.* Cambridge: Cambridge University Press, 1991.

Garnett, A. Campbell. "Conscience and conscientiousness." In *Moral Concepts.* Edited by Joel Feinberg. 80–92. Oxford: Oxford University Press, 1982.

Garvey, John, Mary Ann Glendon, Robert P. George, O. Carter Snead, Yuval Levin, et al. "Unacceptable." www.becketfund.org/wp-content/uploads/2012/04/Unacceptable-4-11.pdf.

Geach, Peter. *The virtues.* Cambridge: Cambridge University Press, 1977.

Geaves, Ron. "Islam and conscience." In *Conscience in world religions.* Edited by Jayne Hoose. 155–75. Notre Dame, IN: University of Notre Dame Press, 1999.

Gehlbach, T. G., L. A. Shinkunas, V. L. Forman-Hoffman, K. W. Thomas, G. A. Schmidt, and L. C. Kaldjian. "Code status orders and goals of care in the medical intensive care unit." *Chest* 139 (2011): 802–809.

Glover, Jonathan. *Humanity: a moral history of the twentieth century.* New Haven, CT: Yale University Press, 1999.

Goldman, Gilbert M. "The tacit dimension of clinical judgment." *Yale Journal of Biology and Medicine* 63 (1990): 47–61.

Gomez-Lobo, Alfonso. *Morality and the human goods: an introduction to natural law.* Washington, DC: Georgetown University Press, 2002.

Gorsky, Jonathan. "Conscience in Jewish tradition." In *Conscience in world religions.* Edited by Jayne Hoose. 129–54. Notre Dame, IN: University of Notre Dame Press, 1999.

Granrose, John T. "The authority of conscience." In *Conscience.* Edited by John Donnelly and Leonard Lyons. 221–35. Staten Island, NY: Alba House, 1973.

Greenawalt, Kent. *Religious convictions and political choice.* New York: Oxford University Press, 1988.

Grisez, Germain, and Russell Shaw. "Conscience: knowledge of moral truth." In *Conscience.* Edited by Charles E. Curran. 39–50. Mahwah, NJ: Paulist Press, 2004.

Gustafson, James M. *Protestant and Roman Catholic ethics: prospects for rapprochement.* Chicago: University of Chicago Press, 1978.

Haberle, T. H., L. A. Shinkunas, Z. D. Erekson, and L. C. Kaldjian. "Goals of care among hospitalized patients: a validation study." *American Journal of Hospice and Palliative Medicine* 28 (2010): 335–41.

Habermas, Jürgen. "Religion in the public sphere." Jürgen Habermas and the Holberg Prize, 2005.

Hafferty, F. W., and R. Franks. "The hidden curriculum, ethics teaching, and the structure of medical education." *Academic Medicine* 69 (1994): 861–71.

Hallowell, John H. "Conscience and civil authority." In *Conscience: its freedom and limitations*. Edited by William C. Bier. 159–69. New York: Fordham University Press, 1971.

Halpern, Jodi. "Clinical empathy in medical care." In *Empathy: from bench to bedside*. Edited by Jean Decety. 229–44. Cambridge, MA: MIT Press, 2012.

Hanson, Mark J., and Daniel Callahan, eds. *The goals of medicine: the forgotten issues in health care reform*. Washington, DC: Georgetown University Press, 1999.

Hardt, John J. "The conscience debate: resources for rapprochement from the problem's perceived source." *Theoretical Medicine and Bioethics* 29 (2008): 151–60.

Harrison, Matthew C., and Samuel Rodriguez. "HHS mandate: an attack on all people of faith." *Washington Post*, August 9, 2012.

Hauerwas, Stanley. "Reconciling the practice of reason: casuistry in a Christian context." In *Moral theory and moral judgments in medical ethics*. Edited by Baruch A. Brody. 135–55. Dordrecht: Kluwer Academic, 1988.

Hebblethwaite, Brian. *Ethics and religion in a pluralistic age*. Edinburgh: T. & T. Clark, 1997.

Hurley, A. C., and L. Volicer. "Alzheimer disease: 'It's okay, Mama, if you want to go, it's okay.'" *JAMA* 288 (2002): 2324–31.

Hursthouse, Rosalind. "Normative virtue ethics." In *Virtue ethics*. Edited by Stephen Darwall. 184–202. Oxford: Blackwell, 2003.

On virtue ethics. Oxford: Oxford University Press, 1999.

Institute of Medicine. *Conflict of interest in medical research, education, and practice*. Washington, DC: National Academies Press, 2009.

Jackson, Philip L., Andrew N. Meltzoff, and Jean Decety. "How do we perceive the pain of others? A window into the neural processes involved in empathy." *NeuroImage* 24 (2005): 771–79.

Jonsen, Albert R. "The therapeutic relationship: is moral conduct a necessary condition?" In *The clinical encounter*. Edited by Earl E. Shelp. 267–87. Dordrecht: Reidel, 1983.

Kaldjian, Lauris C. "Teaching practical wisdom in medicine through clinical judgment, goals of care, and ethical reasoning." *Journal of Medical Ethics* 36 (2010): 558–62.

Kaldjian, Lauris C., Ann E. Curtis, Laura A. Shinkunas, and Katrina T. Cannon. "Goals of care toward the end of life: a structured literature review." *American Journal of Hospice and Palliative Medicine* 25 (2009): 501–11.

Kaldjian, Lauris C., Zachary D. Erekson, Tyler H. Haberle, Ann E. Curtis, Laura A. Shinkunas, Katrina T. Cannon, and Valerie L. Forman-Hoffman. "Code status discussions and goals of care among hospitalized adults." *Journal of Medical Ethics* 35 (2009): 338–42.

Kaldjian, Lauris C., Valerie L. Forman-Hoffman, Elizabeth W. Jones, Barry J. Wu, Benjamin H. Levi, and Gary E. Rosenthal. "Do faculty and resident physicians discuss their medical errors?" *Journal of Medical Ethics* 34 (2008): 717–22.

Kaldjian, Lauris C., Elizabeth W. Jones, Gary E. Rosenthal, Toni Tripp-Reimer, and Stephen Hillis. "An empirically derived taxonomy of factors affecting physicians' willingness to disclose medical errors." *Journal of General Internal Medicine* 21 (2006): 942–48.

Kaldjian, Lauris C., Elizabeth W. Jones, Barry J. Wu, Valerie L. Forman-Hoffman, Benjamin H. Levi, and Gary E. Rosenthal. "Disclosing medical errors to patients: attitudes and practices of physicians and trainees." *Journal of General Internal Medicine* 22 (2007): 988–96.

"Reporting medical errors to improve patient safety: a survey of physicians in teaching hospitals." *Archives of Internal Medicine* 168 (2008): 40–46.

Kaldjian, Lauris C., Laura A. Shinkunas, Mercedes Bern-Klug, and Susan K. Schultz. "Dementia, goals of care, and personhood: a study of surrogate decision makers' beliefs and values." *American Journal of Hospice and Palliative Medicine* 27 (2010): 387–97.

Kant, Immanuel. *Lectures on ethics.* Indianapolis: Hackett, 1963.

Kass, Leon R. "Regarding the end of medicine and the pursuit of health." In *Concepts of health and disease: interdisciplinary perspectives.* Edited by Arthur L. Caplan, H. Tristram Engelhardt, and James J. McCartney. 3–30. London: Addison-Wesley, 1981.

Kassirer, Jerome P., and Richard I. Kopelman. *Learning clinical reasoning.* Baltimore: Williams & Wilkins, 1991.

King, Lester S. "What is disease?" In *Concepts of health and disease: interdisciplinary perspectives.* Edited by Arthur L. Caplan, H. Tristram Engelhardt, and James J. McCartney. 107–18. London: Addison-Wesley, 1981.

Kohn, L. T., J. M. Corrigan, and M. S. Donaldson. *To err is human: building a safer health system.* Washington, DC: National Academy Press, 2000.

Ladd, John. "The internal morality of medicine: an essential dimension of the patient–physician relationship." In *The clinical encounter.* Edited by Earl E. Shelp. 209–31. Dordrecht: Reidel, 1983.

LaFollette, Eva, and Hugh LaFollette. "Private conscience, public acts." *Journal of Medical Ethics* 33 (2007): 249–54.

Langston, Douglas C. *Conscience and other virtues: from Bonaventure to Macintyre.* University Park: Pennsylvania State University Press, 2001.

Lantos, John, Ann Marie Matlock, and David Wendler. "Clinician integrity and limits to patient autonomy." *JAMA* 305 (2011): 495–99.

Lauridsen, Sigurd. "Administrative gatekeeping: a third way between unrestricted patient advocacy and bedside rationing." *Bioethics* 23 (2009): 311–20.

Lawrence, Ryan E., and Farr A. Curlin. "Physicians' beliefs about conscience in medicine: a national survey." *Academic Medicine* 84 (2009): 1276–82.

Lear, Jonathan. *Aristotle: the desire to understand.* Cambridge: Cambridge University Press, 1988.

Little, David. "A view of conscience within the Protestant theological tradition." In *Conscience: its freedom and limitations.* Edited by William C. Bier. 20–28. New York: Fordham University Press, 1971.

Louden, Robert B. "On some vices of virtue ethics." *American Philosophical Quarterly* 21, no. 3 (1984): 227–36.

MacIntyre, Alasdair. *After virtue.* Notre Dame, IN: University of Notre Dame Press, 1984.

"Social structures and their threats to moral agency." *Philosophy* 74 (1995): 311–29.

Maritain, Jacques. *The rights of man and natural law.* New York: Gordian Press, 1971.

Maurer, Christian. "† σύνοιδα, † συνείδησις." In *Theological dictionary of the New Testament.* Edited by Gerhard Kittel and Gerhard Friedrich. 898–919. Grand Rapids, MI: Eerdmans, 1971.

May, Thomas. "Rights of conscience in health care." *Social Theory and Practice* 27 (2001): 111–28.

May, William E. *An introduction to moral theology.* Huntington, IN: Our Sunday Visitor, Inc., 2003.

May, William F. *The physician's covenant: images of the healer in medical ethics.* 2d ed. Louisville: Westminster John Knox Press, 2000.

McCarthy, Joan, and Rick Deady. "Moral distress reconsidered." *Nursing Ethics* 15, no. 2 (2008): 254–62.

McConnell, Michael W. "The origins and historical understanding of free exercise of religion." *Harvard Law Review* 103, no. 7 (1990): 1409–517.

McGuire, Martin C. "On conscience." In *Conscience.* Edited by John Donnelly and Leonard Lyons. 145–57. Staten Island, NY: Alba House, 1973.

McInerny, Ralph. "Ethics." In *Aquinas.* Edited by Norman Kretzmann and Eleonore Stump. 196–216. Cambridge: Cambridge University Press, 1993.

Meilaender, Gilbert C. *The theory and practice of virtue.* Notre Dame, IN: University of Notre Dame Press, 1984.

Miller, William Lee. *Lincoln's virtues: an ethical biography.* New York: Knopf, 2002.

Minow, Martha. "On being a religious professional: the religious turn in professional ethics." *University of Pennsylvania Law Review* 150 (2001): 539–67.

Mitchell, Basil. "The role of theology in bioethics." In *Theology and bioethics.* Edited by E. E. Shelp. 65–78. Dordrecht: Reidel, 1985.

Nagel, Thomas. "The fragmentation of value." In *Knowledge, value and belief.* Edited by H. Tristram Engelhardt and Daniel Callahan. 279–94. Hastings-on-Hudson, NY: Institute of Society, Ethics and the Life Sciences, 1977.

"Moral conflict and political legitimacy." *Philosophy and Public Affairs* 16, no. 3 (1987): 215–40.

Niebuhr, Reinhold. *The children of light and the children of darkness.* New York: Scribner's, 1960.

Nussbaum, L. Martin. "Church v. state: the historic lawsuits over the HHS abortifacient/contraceptive mandate." November 15, 2012. www.preservereligiousfreedom.org/2012/11/church-v-state-the-historic-lawsuits-over-the-hhs-abortifacientcontraceptive-mandate/.

Nussbaum, Martha C. *Liberty of conscience: in defense of America's tradition of religious equality.* New York: Basic Books, 2008.

O'Connell, Laurence J., and Martin E. Marty. "Religious beliefs and bioethics: a crossed relationship." In *Notes from a narrow ridge: religion and bioethics.* Edited by Dena S. Davis and Laurie Zoloth. 215–25. Hagerstown, MD: University Publishing Group, 1999.

O'Reilly, Kevin B. "Doctors advised to consider costs in care choices." *American Medical News*, July 9, 2012.

Owens, Douglas K., Amir Qaseem, Roger Chou, and Paul Shekelle, for the Clinical Guidelines Committee of the American College of Physicians. "High-value, cost-conscious health care: concepts for clinicians to evaluate the benefits, harms, and costs of medical interventions." *Annals of Internal Medicine* 154 (2011): 174–80.

Parsons, Talcott. "Definitions of health and illness in the light of American values and social structure." In *Concepts of Health and Disease: Interdisciplinary Perspectives.* Edited by Arthur L. Caplan, H. Tristram Engelhardt, and James J. McCartney. 57–81. London: Addison-Wesley, 1981.

Pellegrino, Edmund D. "The anatomy of clinical judgments: some notes on right reason and right action." In *Clinical judgment: a critical appraisal.* Edited by H. Tristram Engelhardt, Stuart F. Spicker, and Bernard Towers. 169–94. Dordrecht: Reidel, 1979.

"The goals and ends of medicine: how are they to be defined?" In *Physician & philosopher: the philosophical foundation of medicine – essays by Dr. Edmund Pellegrino.* Edited by Roger J. Bulger and John P. McGovern. 56–65. Charlottesville, VA: Carden Jennings, 2001.

Humanism and the physician. Knoxville: University of Tennessee Press, 1979.

"The physician's conscience, conscience clauses, and religious belief: a Catholic perspective." *Fordham Urban Law Journal* 30 (2002): 221–44.

"The virtuous physician, and the ethics of medicine." In *Virtue and medicine.* Edited by Earl E. Shelp. 237–55. Dordrecht: Reidel, 1985.

Pellegrino, Edmund D., and David C. Thomasma. *A philosophical basis of medical practice: toward a philosophy and ethic of the healing professions.* New York: Oxford University Press, 1981.

The virtues in medical practice. New York: Oxford University Press, 1993.

"Physician's Oath, Declaration of Geneva." World Medical Association. www.wma.net/en/30publications/10policies/g1/

Pieper, Josef. *The four cardinal virtues.* Notre Dame, IN: University of Notre Dame Press, 1966.

Pierce, C. A. *Conscience in the New Testament.* London: SCM Press, 1955.

Pincoffs, Edmund L. "Two cheers for Meno: the definition of the virtues." In *Virtue and medicine.* Edited by Earl E. Shelp. 111–31. Dordrecht: Reidel, 1985.

Plantinga, Alvin. "Reason and belief in God." In *Faith and rationality: reason and belief in God.* Edited by Alvin Plantinga and Nicholas Wolterstorff. 16–93. Notre Dame, IN: University of Notre Dame Press, 1983.

Ramsey, Paul. *Ethics at the edges of life.* Eugene, OR: Wipf & Stock, 2000.

Ratzinger, Joseph. *On conscience.* San Francisco: Ignatius Press, 2007.

Rawls, John. "The idea of public reason revisited." *University of Chicago Law Review* 64, no. 3 (1997): 765–807.

Justice as fairness: a restatement. Edited by Erin Kelly. Cambridge, MA: Harvard University Press, 2001.

Political liberalism. New York, NY: Columbia University Press, 1993.

"Political liberalism and religion." Yale University, October 6–7, 1994.

A theory of justice. Cambridge, MA: Harvard University Press, 1971.

Reeder, John P. "The dependence of ethics." In *James M. Gustafson's theocentric ethics: interpretations and assessments.* Edited by Harlan R. Beckley and Charles M. Swezey. 119–41. Macon, GA: Mercer University Press, 1988.

"What is a religious ethic?" *Journal of Religious Ethics* 25, no. 3 (suppl. S) (1998): 157–81.

Rothman, D. J., and S. C. Chimonas. "New developments in managing physician–industry relationships." *JAMA* 300 (2008): 1067–69.

Savulescu, Julian. "Conscientious objection in medicine." *British Medical Journal* 332 (2006): 294–97.

Schafer, Arthur. "Bedside rationing by physicians: the case against." *Healthcare Papers* 2 (2001): 45–52.

Scriven, Michael. "Clinical judgment." In *Clinical judgment: a critical appraisal,* edited by H. Tristram Engelhardt, Stuart F. Spicker, and Bernard Towers. 3–16. Dordrecht: Reidel, 1979.

Shapiro, Johanna. "The paradox of teaching empathy in medical education." In *Empathy: from bench to bedside.* Edited by Jean Decety. 275–90. Cambridge, MA: MIT Press, 2012.

Siegler, Mark. "The doctor–patient encounter and its relationship to theories of health and disease." In *Concepts of health and disease: interdisciplinary perspectives.* Edited by Arthur L. Caplan, H. Tristram Engelhardt, and James J. McCartney. 627–44. London: Addison-Wesley, 1981.

Singer, P. A., S. R. Benatar, M. Bernstein, A. S. Daar, B. M. Dickens, S. K. MacRae, R. E. G. Upshur, L. Wright, and R. Z. Shaul. "Ethics and SARS: lessons from Toronto." *British Medical Journal* 327 (2003): 1342–44.

Smart, J. J. C., and Bernard Williams. *Utilitarianism: for and against.* Cambridge: Cambridge University Press, 1973.

Smart, Ninian. "Religion." In The Westminster dictionary of Christian theology. Edited by Alan Richardson and John Bowden. 496–98. Philadelphia: Westminster Press, 1983.

Smith, Cynthia D. "Teaching high-value, cost-conscious care to residents: the Alliance for Academic Internal Medicine–American College of Physicians curriculum." *Annals of Internal Medicine* 157 (2012): 284–86.

Snyder, Lois, and Daniel P. Sulmasy. "Physician-assisted suicide (American College of Physicians position paper)." *Annals of Internal Medicine* 135 (2001): 209–16.

Sober, Elliott. "The art and science of clinical judgment: an informational approach." In *Clinical judgment: a critical appraisal.* Edited by H. Tristram Engelhardt, Stuart F. Spicker, and Bernard Towers. 29–44. Dordrecht: Reidel, 1979.

Spohn, William C. "Conscience and moral development." In *Conscience.* Edited by Charles E. Curran. 130–50. Mahwah, NJ: Paulist Press, 2004.

Stallings, Destyn D. "A tough pill to swallow: whether the Patient Protection and Affordable Care Act obligates Catholic organizations to cover their employees' prescription contraceptives." *Tulsa Law Review* 48 (2012): 117–41.

Stout, Jeffrey. *Ethics after Babel: the languages of morals and their discontents.* Princeton, NJ: Princeton University Press, 2001.

Sullivan, W. M. "Medicine under threat: professionalism and professional identity." *Canadian Medical Association Journal* 162 (2000): 673–75.

Sulmasy, Daniel P. "What is conscience and why is respect for it so important?" *Theoretical Medicine and Bioethics* 29 (2008): 201–12.

Swick, Herbert M. "Toward a normative definition of medical professionalism." *Academic Medicine* 75 (2000): 612–16.

Taylor, Charles. "The diversity of goods." In *Utilitarianism and beyond*. Edited by Amartya Sen and Bernard Williams. 129–44. Cambridge: Cambridge University Press, 1982.

The ethics of authenticity. Cambridge, MA: Harvard University Press, 1991.

Sources of the self. Cambridge, MA: Harvard University Press, 1989.

Thomas, Stephen. "Conscience in Orthodox thought." In *Conscience in world religions*. Edited by Jayne Hoose. 99–125. Notre Dame, IN: University of Notre Dame Press, 1999.

Tillich, Paul. *Dynamics of faith*. New York: Harper & Row, 1957.

Ubell, Peter A. "Physicians, thou shalt ration: the necessary role of bedside rationing in controlling healthcare costs." *Healthcare Papers* 2 (2001): 10–21.

United States House of Representatives. H.R. 1179: Respect for Rights of Conscience Act of 2011.

Veatch, Robert M. "The sources of professional ethics: why professions fail." *Lancet* 373 (2009): 1000–1001.

Walley, R. "A question of conscience." *British Medical Journal* 1 (1976): 1456–58.

Walzer, Michael. *Thick and thin: moral argument at home and abroad*. Notre Dame, IN: University of Notre Dame Press, 1994.

Wand, Bernard. "The content and function of conscience." In *Conscience*. Edited by John Donnelly and Leonard Lyons. 133–43. Staten Island, NY: Alba House, 1973.

Wardle, Lynn D. "Protecting the rights of conscience of health care providers." *Journal of Legal Medicine* 14 (1993): 177–230.

White, Katherine A. "Crisis of conscience: reconciling religious health care providers' beliefs and patients' rights." *Stanford Law Review* 51 (1999): 1703–49.

Wicclair, Mark R. *Conscientious objection in health care: an ethical analysis*. Cambridge: Cambridge University Press, 2011.

"Conscientious objection in medicine." *Bioethics* 14 (2000): 205–27.

Williams, Bernard. *Moral luck*. Cambridge: Cambridge University Press, 1981.

Wilson, Robin Fretwell. "The limits of conscience: moral clashes over deeply divisive healthcare procedures." *American Journal of Law & Medicine* 34 (2008): 41–63.

Wolterstorff, Nicholas. "Can belief in God be rational if it has no foundations?" In *Faith and rationality: reason and belief in God*. Edited by Alvin Plantinga and Nicholas Wolterstorff. 135–86. Notre Dame, IN: University of Notre Dame Press, 1983.

Wynia, M. K., S. R. Latham, A. C. Kao, J. W. Berg, and L. L. Emanuel. "Medical professionalism in society." *New England Journal of Medicine* 341 (1999): 1612–16.

Young, Michael J., Sydney E. S. Brown, Robert D. Truog, and Scott D. Halpern. "Rationing in the intensive care unit: to disclose or disguise?" *Critical Care Medicine* 40 (2012): 261–66.

Zachman, Randall C. *The assurance of faith: conscience in the theology of Martin Luther and John Calvin*. Louisville: Westminster John Knox Press, 2005.

Index